AGING ISSUES, HEALTH AND FINANCIAL ALTERNATIVES

ELDERLY PATIENTS WITH MULTI-MORBIDITY, FRAILTY AND GERIATRIC SYNDROMES: THERAPEUTIC PROBLEM OF CONTEMPORARY AND INCOMING MEDICINE AT INTENSIVE CARE UNIT (ICU) FROM THE GERIATRICIAN'S VIEWPOINT

AGING ISSUES, HEALTH AND FINANCIAL ALTERNATIVES

Additional books in this series can be found on Nova's website under the Series tab.

Additional E-books in this series can be found on Nova's website under the E-books tab.

AGING ISSUES, HEALTH AND FINANCIAL ALTERNATIVES

ELDERLY PATIENTS WITH MULTI-MORBIDITY, FRAILTY AND GERIATRIC SYNDROMES: THERAPEUTIC PROBLEM OF CONTEMPORARY AND INCOMING MEDICINE AT INTENSIVE CARE UNIT (ICU) FROM THE GERIATRICIAN'S VIEWPOINT

PAVEL WEBER

Nova Science Publishers, Inc.
New York

NOTICE TO THE READER

LIBRARY OF CONGRESS CATALOGING-IN-PUBLICATION DATA
Weber, Pavel.
Elderly patients with multi-morbidity, frailty, and geriatric syndromes :
therapeutic problem of contemporary and incoming medicine at intensive care
unit (ICU) from the geriatrician's viewpoint / Pavel Weber.
p. ; cm.
Includes bibliographical references and index.
ISBN 978-1-61761-176-6 (softcover)
1. Older people--Diseases. 2. Aging--Physiological aspects. 3.
Comorbidity. I. Title.
[DNLM: 1. Geriatrics. 2. Aging--physiology. 3. Comorbidity. 4. Frail
Elderly. 5. Intensive Care. WT 100]
RC952.5W43 2010
618.97--dc22
2010028493

Published by Nova Science Publishers, Inc. ✢ New York

CONTENTS

PREFACE

The chapter aims at presenting a practically orientated survey of major problems of a clinical picture and therapeutic pitfalls in critically ill elderly patients from the point of view of a geriatrician. Growing number of the patients of advanced age represent a highly heterogeneous group with very different health problems. For the ICU admitted elderly patients are valuable general pitfalls of modern medicine connected with: atomization of medicine; absence of holistic approach and contemporary multi-morbidity when they belong to miscellaneous medical branches according to principal somatic diagnosis or seemingly nowhere.

It is obvious that the intensivist should acquire at least basic knowledge of geriatric problems to enhance their knowledge of multi-morbidity, frailty and geriatric syndromes and their interrelationships. The management and treatment of factual somatic status and disease of critically ill elderly persons in ICU is always connected with potential undesirable effect of therapy on frail older person.

Moreover in advanced age typical multi-morbidity is connected with geriatric giants (instability with falls, immobility, incontinence, intellectual and sensual impairments, dehydration etc.). The risk of sudden deterioration of geriatric syndromes with elevated risk of development of delirium, dehydration, malnutrition etc. grows with age substantially.

The potential risk of impairment in senior patients is much more serious than in younger ones because of further independence problems. Overall treatment of any disease in advanced age (including geriatric syndromes and frailty) should be aimed not only at causing disease but also protection and/or improvement of self-sufficiency, functioning social relations in family and community.

In clinical practice every patient should be assessed individually at admission to ICU. Possibilities of therapeutic efforts in advanced age will be limited by physical and mental abilities and the senior's social environment. Optimal intensive treatment of the elderly should remove symptoms of the disease, achieve sufficient compensation of somatic status and prevent from complications. The significant part of the ICU hospitalized patients are people of advanced age (between 25-50%). Their hospital stay in ICU is longer in comparison to younger people. It is envisaged that this share will grow according to the demographic prognosis. Therefore it becomes essential for any intensivist to familiarise with fundamental gerontologic problems.

The main goal of geriatric medicine valuable also for the area of intensive care is:

1. retain the health of seniors
2. enable them to live qualitatively and independently as long as possible
3. minimize period with frailty syndrome

Keywords: Advanced age – multi-morbidity – geriatric syndromes – frailty – poly-pharmacy –dehydration – delirium – thermoregulatory disorders

Chapter 1

INTRODUCTION

The development of civilization leads to increasing hope of longer survival and makes the average life expectancy longer. Both in absolute and relative numbers the amount of the elderly, very old and long-aged people are increasing [11,86]. This tendency will continue and it will be emphasized by ageing volumes of people born after the World War 2 in the years 2010 -2015 [52]. The basic survey and knowledge of geriatric medicine will be necessary in the future, especially for professionals such as doctors, nurses, psychologists, social workers, physio- and occupational therapists etc.

The old age life is not easy and there are many exposures – health problems, loneliness, misunderstandings, loss of advisability, self – sufficiency and autonomy, poverty, age segregation and discrimination (ageism).

This chapter is dealing with specific care of critically ill patients of old age and it is showing some of the important points in geriatrics, which are very close to intensive medicine and generally to problems of medicine in care of advanced age population [18,27,37]. The main problems of modern and internally differentiated medicine in care of senior population are:

1. atomization of medicine
2. absence of holistic approach
3. multi-morbidity - it means it does not belong to any or many specializations
4. enormous socialization of health problems

On the contrary there is significantly higher need of long-term hospitalization in case of multi-morbid seniors [39,119], who demand specific procedures, attitude and knowledge of the doctors. Numerous prospective studies [20,88,89] show that old-aged patients gain from hospitalization on specialized intensive geriatric wards (less complications, re-hospitalizations etc.) Moreover, the expenses are lowered. Knowledge of at least basic extraordinarities and specifics of geriatric medicine will be of huge practical significance, because in the year 2050 there will live 2 billions of people older that 60 years on the Earth. [74]. From this fact it is obvious, that there is an objective need to master the basic knowledge of gerontology and geriatrics among professionals (including intensivists).

In this brief chapter it is not possible to include the whole issue dealing with the intensive care and stay of old-aged patients on ICU, even if this issue deserves the attention because of its practical meaning and close relationship with other branches (internal medicine, surgery etc.). The emergency situations together with polymorbidity and exhaustion of functional reserves in advanced age [20,36] will be more frequent in all of the organ systems – cardiovascular, respiratory, GI (gastrointestinal) tract, endocrine, immune etc. [12,90]. We refer to the study of the clinical picture description (incl.therapy) of each of critical states in the old age in appropriate specialized chapters in this monograph and in other gerontologic literature [43,105]. We will deal in details with syndromes of delirium, dehydration (incl.mineral balance), disturbance of thermoregulation, when external influences can cause hypothermia or hyperthermia. We suppose that these states are very important and very frequent in old age and with which they are directly connected. Because of these reasons we pay special attention to this issue in this chapter.

General knowledge of these aspects can substantially influence an approach of intensivists who face an increasing number of old patients in their practice [17,79]. Among the aspects we would like to mention there are: global situation, specific problem of geriatric medicine, pharmacotherapy in the elderly, at last but not least problems of ageing organism as reflected in particularities and pitfalls of ICU treatment in multi-morbid old patients, especially risks of drug interactions which is highly topical in these people for their poly-pharmacotherapy if anyone is interested in deeper studies of geriatric medicine problems we can refer them to appropriate monographs and textbooks listed in the references [21,77]. Generally acute severity of illness in the elderly is even more strongly associated with mortality. Consequently, age alone may be an inappropriate criterion for allocation of ICU resources.

Ageing and its manifestation as currently understood such as frailty, functional disorders and decreasing mental abilities are not standard symptoms of ageing process but they are mostly consequences of simultaneously ongoing diseases [41,53]. The target of new *interventional gerontology is extension of active life period and sustaining functional abilities for maximum time.*

Geriatric medicine seeks to achieve maximum sustainability of appropriate physical and mental activities, prevention from self-sufficiency loss and improvement of older people expectations in case they fall ill. It is orientated to *intervention and prevention and supports successful healthy ageing* [107]. It is not nursing or terminal care which should be understood as a chief aim of modern geriatrics which on the contrary concentrates on management of diseases with modified clinical picture and consequential social problems of the elderly.

Growing number of elderly patients in last decades and considerably small awareness of this fact in wider medical public makes this chapter highly significant. It is obvious that intensivists should acquire at least basic knowledge of geriatric problems to enhance their knowledge of critically ill old age people in order to improve their management in ICU [111].

Chapter 2

Clinical Gerontology and Comprehensive Geriatric Assessment (CGA)

Clinical gerontology or geriatry is a special medical branch of interdisciplinary character. The object of interest is ageing and old person sane and especially insane. It deals with many particularities of diseases in old age and with their consequences; it is focused on prevention, diagnosis, therapy, physiotherapy and nursing care in pathological forms of ageing and old age [83]. It uses specific methods and forms of work; it deals with chronic conditions connected with loss of functional potential, with waning of self-sufficiency and increasing of dependence. [112]. This branch is in close connection with other medical branches and integrates their knowledge about the old and disordered persons.

Clinical gerontology emphasizes an individual approach to old patients [9,104]. The method of operation is *comprehensive geriatric assessment* - CGA [42,83,117]. Apart from somatic aspects of the health status there are significant items to be underlined: self-sufficiency evaluation, knowledge and evaluation of psychic state and social conditions (see table 1.).

In its multidisciplinary context the geriatry does not substitute other clinical medical branches in care of an old person but completes them with application of *specific geriatric regimen*, which aims to reinforce the independence and improve self-sufficiency of the older patients [117].

Table 1. Comprehensive geriatric assessment

Subject of assessment	Way of evaluation
Somatic status	Somatic examination, posture, mobility, continence, nutrition, sight, hearing, geriatric syndromes, etc.
Self-sufficiency	ADL- test, ability to keep own household, IADL-test
Mental status	cognitive function – MMSE- test, Clock test; depression scale according Yesavage, etc.
Social status	social contacts, people available to summon help, bereavement, removal, dwelling and loneliness risks

Following methods are based on principles of *specific geriatric regimen.*

- Considerate tailor-made diagnostics and treatment aimed at improvement of life quality
- Follow up physiotherapy
- Multi-disciplinary team active approach aimed at improvement of self-sufficiency and/or prevention of dependence
- Social work creating conditions enabling patients to return to home environment (incl. home-care)

Main target of these efforts is improvement in independence and self-sufficiency improvement in older patients. Geriatric regimen brings benefits especially for patients aged 75+ or even 80+ who are endangered with following risks typical for this age:

- ➢ Development of immobilisation syndrome
- ➢ Self-sufficiency loss
- ➢ Atypical pathway of more diseases influencing simultaneously each other
- ➢ Occurrence of early impairment of organ function as a consequence of exhaustion of their functional reserve (lungs, kidneys etc.)
- ➢ Maladaptation towards changes
- ➢ Ageism (discrimination because of the old age).

Chapter 3

GERIATRIC PATIENT – PARTICULARITIES

Geriatric patients are people of higher age (formally above 65; practically above 75 years), their involutionary and morbid changes (usually multi-morbidity) significantly influenced their functional state, adaptability, ability of regulation, toleration to stress. These patients profit from specific geriatric attitude, they need more complicated coordination of services, often active observation of health and/or functional state, they are in risk of sudden loss of self-sufficiency, danger of delay, adverse effect of remedies is more frequent, institutional care is often needed (geriatric hospitalism), also they are in danger of frequent professional mistakes for atypical symptoms in comparison to clinical picture, which is for certain disease typical in adult middle age [79,117].

Geriatric patients differ from the others in the way of interpretation of his/her etiopathogenetic diagnosis assessed with classical biomedical methods which normally does not tell us how extensive care is needed, in what ways he or she becomes dependent on his/her environment and how and where they can live their future life [35,106]. Treatment of the elderly (especially in late advanced age) cannot be aimed exclusively at managing the essential disease, which can be sometimes impossible, but it should be orientated towards maintenance and/or improvement of self-sufficiency and functioning social relations and contacts within the family and the community in general [106].

Majority of all biological functions culminates before the age of 30 y. Some of them gradually continuously decrease afterwards [70]. This decay is practically of no significance in terms of current everyday activity but it can matter under stress or extended load [47, 48].

Seniors as such represent very heterogenous group and from the point of view of fitness, risk and need of help (or specific service) they can be divided to the 3 basic areas with different focus of health attention:

- *Fit seniors* – Seniors in good condition and physical efficiency. Medical attitude towards them should be the same as standards which are valid for adults in middle age. However, there can be also risk of atypical symptoms of diseases in them.
- *Independent seniors* – do not need extraordinary care and services, they can live independently in standard condition, however in stress situations (severe diseases, surgery, injuries, viral infections in epidemies, extreme variation of the weather, sudden change of social state – death of partner, loneliness, moving etc.) they fail.
- *Frail seniors* – are instable and in the risk even in standard condition. These frail seniors usually need help in common daily activities or they are limited in motion, moreover they can be confined to bed [34,115]. This group of patients contains those with higher risk of falls, dementia syndrome, with very bad mobility, labile somatic disease (i.e. frail cardiac with repeated cardiac failure or electric instability), also with complicated orientation (visual disturbance and hearing loss), people in social distress and very old above 85 years old, especially when they live alone [65,122].

Chapter 4

BIOLOGY OF AGEING

Ageing and advanced age is a terminal phase of ontogenetic development of every individual [9,79]. *Specific degenerative morphological* and *functional changes* occur in individual organs at all levels from the cells to whole organism [45]. Important role in ageing is *apoptosis* [59]. In the cell, which may compromise the body (eg, activated leukocyt, as malignant cells), respectively a correction would be difficult to run programmed cell death.

This happens in different periods of times and in different speed. It affects any living substance from the moment of it's birth (conception). The life expectancy of an individual in nature is generically specific and has important inter-individual variability. Ageing speed of an individual is genetically coded – it is presumed that this *type of genetics is a multi-factorial one* [70]. Maximum potential life expectancy of a human being attainable under ideal circumstances could be 110 - 120 y. The influence of genetic factor on the life expectancy is considered about 35 per cent. The resting 65 per cent represent an influence of a life style and external environment.

Common and typical features of ageing in general:

1. loss of functional parenchyma of individual organs = *involution*
2. decay of physical performance, deteriorated regeneration after load and reduced tolerance towards load
3. influence of one or more diseases
4. disintegrated ageing: big inter- and intra-individual differences (organs and systems)
5. effort to create new own homeostatic mechanisms (which accompanies growing involution) = *adaptability*.

The answer to the question why we get old is in *theories of ageing*. There are plenty of them and it is not rare that the cause and the consequence are swapped by mistake [70,79]. The speculation about the most important mechanism is concerned mainly in two questions: if the process is programmed, determined or if it is random, stochastic. The most known theories can be distinguished into two main groups: a) those, which suppose that the processes connected with ageing are random and with the age is growing the disturbance and failure of cell conduction = *stochastic theory* ; b) those, which say, that the ageing is determined by genetic information = *non-stochastic theory.*

Senile performance decline is a consequence [9] of general weakness, impaired locomotion and balance, lower stamina. The life expectancy is significantly influenced by risk factors, contingent metabolic changes and level of resistance to stress. A choice of life style is also essential. Ageing in human population is often connected with increased occurrence of degenerative affections, tumours and Alzheimer's disease.

In fact it should be a period of life in which broad harmonic development of human personality goes on and on. Most people of advanced age should remain independent, self-sufficient and retaining their good psychic condition up to the terminal period of their life.

Chapter 5

DEMOGRAPHIC ANALYSIS OF CONTEMPORARY AND FUTURAL WORLD POPULATION

In the beginning of the 20th century 3 to 5 per cent of population in European industrial countries (similarly in USA) were people aged 65+ y. This percentage has grown up to 14 – 20 % nowadays. Up to the fifties of previous century people died prematurely. During the last hundred years the life expectancy (LE) almost doubled which is one of the greatest achievements of mankind and science in general. Length of human life begins to approach to its biological limit. Probability of achieving advanced age is no longer exceptional, on the contrary it becomes a standard [53,79,86].

Absolute and relative growth of number of the elderly both in developed and developing countries is a main feature of population development in the 21st century [98]. We speak about *population ageing*. There are approx. 580 mil. people aged 60+ in the today's world out of which 355 mil. live in developing countries. In 2050 there will be 2 billions of our planet inhabitants aged 60+ y. This age category will overweight children of < 14 y. The most rapid increase during the next decades is envisaged in the 80+ y. group in the industrial countries. It is the ageing of old population [19]. In the USA, Canada and majority of European union countries it has been found that the most rapidly increasing group of population is the one of 85+ y. (Figure 1).

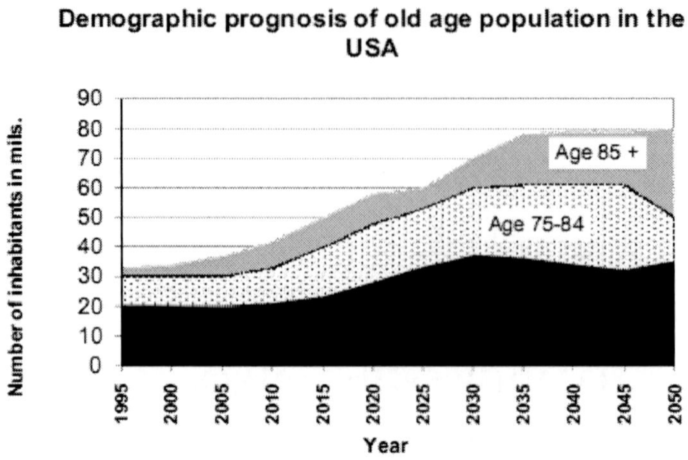

Figure 1. Demographic prognosis of old age population in the USA.

Ageing in the industrial (developed) *countries* can be considered:

- prevailingly gradual
- connected with birth rate decrease
- a consequence of improving life conditions after the industrial revolution
- progress in medicine

In the *developing countries* on the other hand:

- ageing is more rapid
- birth rate decrease is dramatic
- life expectancy grows as a consequence of improving medical care
- ageing leads to enhanced poverty

In 2020 there will be 1 billion of people aged 60+ all over the world which is twice as many as today. 700 mil. of them will live in the developing countries. The highest proportion of these elderly is envisaged in Japan (31 per cent), than in Greece and Switzerland (28 per cent), USA (23 per cent), etc.

The growth of population aged 65+ in Europe and Northern America during the next 30 years is estimated to reach 22 – 30 per cent. Growing number of the elderly brings also both absolute and relative increase of occurrence of affections which are typical for the advanced age and this becomes a serious worldwide social problem [99]. This covers not only typically somatic diseases such as atherosclerosis, cardio- and cerebrovascular events, heart failure, peripheral vasculopathies, parkinsonism, hypo-thyreosis, diabetes, osteoporosis and osteoarthrosis, diverticulosis, anemias, etc. but also mental diseases with all manifestations and consequences of dementia, especially the Alzheimer's type [15,101].

Analogically to the population ageing in society also medical science has experienced a phenomenon of the so called "*geriatrisation of medicine*" which means a significant prevalence of the elderly among all the patients to be treated [4]. This aspect penetrates practically all the branches of medicine to begin with the front line up to the various special fields including ophtalmology.

Chapter 6

CHARACTERISTICS OF AGEING

The elderly are highly heterogeneous group, and individuals become more dissimilar as they age. Individuals over 65 years – with or without chronic diseases – vary widely in their physical, behavioral, and cognitive functions.

The *ageing – is an inevitable physiological process, which is the last ontogenetic period of the human life.* People mostly achieve their old age without any enormous problems. They live to their *„successful ageing"*. in quite comfortable physical, psychical and social balance [28,117]. The somatic (diseases), psychical (dementia, depression) and social (loneliness) problems begin to appear apparently after 75th year (more in women) [5]

The old age and the disease cannot be considered the same thing no matter how often it happens in both non-professional and professional community. In most cases the individual in old age is self-sufficient and fit until the last period of his/her life (many times until the last days). The dependence on care of the others comes with the disease, which can be both somatic and psychical. In between 65 and 75 years nearly 85% of people do not suffer from any significant modifying or common life restricting disease. Even in the age above 85 years 40% of the elderly can live self-sufficiently their normal life [39].

Women live usually 7 – 8 years longer than men [107]. The explanation can be found most likely in gender specific genetic factors and also in biological factors of the environment. The differences in surviving between genders has not changed even in contemporary era, when women smoke more often than ever before and perform originally male professions.

In gerontology we speak sometimes about the so-called *male overmortality*. The consequence of this phenomenon is increasing number of widows as the age increases. This is the base for the typical phenomenon in gerontology – the phenomenon of lonely old women. That fact indirectly increases the consumption of both institutional and non-institutional care in the health and social sphere.

The beginning of the *social old age* is usually seen in the moment of entitlement to regular retirement or the actual retirement [11,119]. The classification of the human age in social sphere is as follows: *the first age* (before productive age, childhood and youth, learning, preparation for profession, acquisition of social experience), *the second age* (productive age, adulthood, biological productivity – breeding, economical and social productivity), *the third age* (post-productive, the old age), eventually *the fourth age* (the period of dependence), which does not take place in every person inevitably. The calendar age is uniquely determined but does not reflect the individual differences of the real health status among the human beings.

The determination of the age zones for the old age is conventional and it is a social frame outgoing from the administrative needs of the social state. In the demographic statistics it is usually worked with the border of 60 or 65 years. Nowadays the beginning of the old age is thought 65 years and the old age itself is considered from 75 years on. From this pattern also the most used division of the old age results:

- *65 – 74 years* old belong to group of *young seniors*, the main problem is the retirement, the free time, activities, self-fulfillment.
- *75 – 84 years, the old seniors,* the problem of adaptability, toleration to stress, specific ailment, loneliness. The *age above 75 years*, when the old age begins in the strict sense of the word, it seems to be break point of ontogenesis, when more significant changes connected with physiological ageing proceed.
- *85 and more years very old aged seniors* („oldest old“) – they are segregated as an individual cathegory for the high occurence of frail seniors and high risk of sudden rise of dependence.

Chapter 7

SOME SPECIFICS OF GERIATRIC MEDICINE

Health status in ageing is a result of many factors, including the chronic diseases of ageing and many other prevalent conditions that cannot be defined as classic „diseases“ because they do not result from a single pathologic cause. Many of the problems affecting aged individuals should be viewed as geriatric syndromes (GS), that are a collection of signs and symptoms with a number of potential causes [44]. Only nowadays the causes and effective treatments of these conditions are beginning to be understood.

In spite of indisputable significance of the atypical clinical picture of diseases in the old age, the *crux of geriatric medicine* is involutionary conditioned *decline of health potential, frailty* and *related geriatric syndromes* and *function deficiency* with their multi-causal reasons. This status is connected with exhaustion of organ reservoirs – "*homeostenosis*". Geriatric syndrome is different from the convenient meaning of the word "syndrome" in clinical medicine, where the symptoms are typical for certain disease [44,49,79]. For the geriatric syndromes numerous and various causes are typical which lead to the occurrence of geriatric syndrome at the end. *Geriatric syndromology* is an essential component of the so-called comprehensive geriatric assessment (CGA) which is extended over the clinical examination in younger non-geriatric population [42,83,117].

Geriatric giants [77,79,107] as geriatric syndromes (GS):

- *immobility* (pressure sore etc.),
- *instability* (dizziness, posture and gait disorders, falls),
- *incontinence,*
- *intellectual disorders* (delirium, dementia and depression),

- *iatrogenia* (dangerous polypharmacy).

They are characterized by their:

A. Multi-causality
B. Chronic course
C. Reduced independence
D. Demanding care and difficult curability

As further geriatric syndromes are respected [44,49]:

- syndrom of hypomobility, decondition and sarcopenia
- anorexia syndrom and malnutrition
- syndrom of dual combined sensoric deficiency (visual and hearing)
- syndrom of dehydration with subsequent manifestation of acute renal failure
- syndrom of thermoregulatory disturbance
- syndrom of elder abuse, neglect and self-neglect sy
- syndrom of geriatric maladaptation
- syndrom of terminal geriatric deterioration - FTT („failure to thrive")

The above mentioned geriatric syndromes not always threaten patient's life but they essentially influence quality of their following life [53,96]. Patients become fully dependent on other people´s assistance (family, friends, neighbours, community services). Not exceptionally they must be admitted to an institutional care (hospitals, nursing homes etc.) because of domestic care system failure or necessity to manage an acute phase of a disease. The expression of the concept of geriatric syndromes in the last decades is a very fundamental step forward in geriatric medicine. The marked part of multi-morbid disabled handicapped seniors can be better understood and earlier and effectively solved (117). GS are more complicated problem with inner connections very often. Their proper identification is made possible by:

- screening tests and observation
- optimalisation of geriatric hospital regime
- optimal coordination of community and institutional services
- influence on anorexia by adjustment of nutrition (proteins 1.3g/kg)
- psychotherapeutical support with elimination of the depression
- lasting physiotherapy (everyday walking at least for 30 minutes)

- attempting to influence the disinterest and weariness by interesting daily activity
- using all of the occupational utilities, which can minimise the dependence (walker, rods, crutches, wheelchairs and other – glasses, magnifying glass, hearing aids
- recondition programs
- adjustment of the living (lightning, grab handles on toilet and corridors, the correct hight of the bed and furniture)

The involutionary loss of muscle tissue in the old age is called *sarcopenia* and it is characterized by reduction of muscle tissue, reduction of the force, tenacity, plasticity and speed of contraction [93]. The probable cause of sarcopenia in senium [94] is apart from somatopausis (lowered level of anabolic IGF-1, growth hormone and testosterone) also influence of oxidatory stress and free radicals produced by muscle mitochondrias [70]. The metabolic result of sarcopenia in the old age is also impaired glucose tolerance and higher risk of diabetes of 2nd type [53,102].

The meaningful concept which is tightly connected with ageing is *frailty* [36,91,120]. This belongs to key characteristics of geriatric patients, the next milestone and the keystone of geriatric medicine. Frailty is a biologic syndrome of decreased reserves in multiple systems that results from dysregulation that can occur with ageing and is initiated by physiological changes of ageing, disease, and/or lack of activity or inadequate nutritional intake.

It is rather more multidimensional concept than just the expression of a degree of dependence in the everyday life activities. Frailty is basically connected with the grow of fatal somatic ailments and lowering of functional reserve of the old person, which is wasting away excessively without any fundamental cause disease. *Frailty* can be defined as a status of reduced physiological reserves connected with increased inclination towards invalidisation (falls, fractures, daily life restrictions, loss of independence) [65,114]. Apart from the clinical observations there is elevation of CRP, leukocytes (monocytes), IL-6, IL-1 and TNF. Frailty is not the synonym of multi-morbidity or disability, multi-morbidity can cause this and disability can be the consequence [34].

Frailty is understood mainly as a risk of sudden deterioration of the status of very risky person. (above 80 years, living alone or with handicapped spouse, with serious somatic or psychical disease). The outcome for those defined frail seniors is the long term need of help of institutions and community (nursing service). The risks of the development of frailty [35,106] are represented by hypomobility in pre-senium, social isolation, depression, bad subjective feeling of the own health etc.

The concept of frailty is at least coming nearer to the term risky geront, used in the past. The emphasis is put on the retrieval of these people because they can not show their frailty out. Both (the ageing and physical frailty) are conditioned by the decline of proteosynthesis in the muscles, decline of immune function, elevation of the mass of fat in the body and lowering of the amount of body water, lowering of the bone mineral density, loss of the whole body mass and strength.

The main etiological and patogenetic mechanisms [65,114] of the syndrome of frailty are:

- the inflammation or hypercoagulation
- oxidative stress
- insuline resistence
- anorexia with loosing of the weight and malnutrition
- sarcopenia
- decline of efficiency of lower extremities
- loosing of spontaneous action – nutrition, hydration, movement, behavioral and social
- dysfunction of autonomic nervous system (falls, sarcopenia, decubital ulcer and healing – with the consequence like loosing the weight, incontinence, delirium, disturbance in thermoregulation etc.)
- apathy – as the consequence of lack of the dopamine in CNS (depression, dementia)
- depression, anxious status, organic psychosyndrome
- development of cognitive deficiency
- menopausis and andropausis as the consequence of hormone deficiency with the development of the syndrome ADAM and PADAM, somatopausis as the result of lack of IGF-1
- chronical pain
- hypomobility with the sedentary lifestyle
- chronic stress
- functionally important consequences of chronic diseases limiting in any activity (hemiparesis, severe diabetic neuropathy, respiratory or heart insufficiency, severe anemia of chronic diseases)
- adverse effects of the medicaments

Chapter 8

IATROGENIA VERSUS POLYPHARMACY

There are several reasons for the greater incidence of iatrogenic drug reactions in the elderly population, the most important of which is the high number of medications that are taken by the elderly, especially those with multiple comorbidities [11,28]. Older individuals often have varying responses to a given serum drug level. Thus, they are more sensitive to some drugs (eg opioids) and less sensitive to others (eg. beta-blockers).

Following aspects should be considered in the old-age pharmacotherapy [54]:

1. Responses to drugs are different from preceeding age categories which is a consequence of changed pharmaco-dynamics and pharmaco-kinetics.
2. Increased occurrence of undesired effects of drugs in general
3. Increased non-compliance in the elderly
4. Increased occurrence of drug interactions

Multi-morbidity of advanced age often leads a physician in clinical practice to *polypharmacotherapy* [77,104], which is many times inevitable but still is sometimes hazardous because with increasing age an occurrence of undesired drug effects grows. The elderly are generally more vulnerable and the therapeutic range gets narrower. Compliance decreases inter-individual variability of an effect increases the same way as the risk of drug interactions. Basic requirement for phamacotherapy in advanced age is that it should be simple, purposeful and effective. Polypharmacy can be often risky and ineffective, many times it can be even damaging – *iatrogenia* as a syndrome.

In geriatric medicine generally symptomatic treatment overweights the causal one. Its undesired effects can substantially alter the clinical picture of diseases.

Drugs in an organism effect simultaneously influencing each other. Such *drug interactions* can change biological response of the organism as a whole in terms of both quantity and quality [66,68]. They belong to drug risks in clinical practice and they can be adverse consequence of combined therapy. Their number grows exponentially with increasing number of administered drugs. They happen at both pharmaco-kinetic and pharmaco-dynamic levels. Drugs can interfere also with some foodstuff (absorption, bio-transformation). Clinical equivalent of risky drug interactions can be hypoglycaemia, haemorrhage, cardiac dysrhythmia, centrally conditioned spasms, blood pressure changes. All these can be triggered by: oral antidiabetics, antidysrhythmics, anticoagulants, psychopharmacs, antiepeleptics etc.

The consumption of drugs in the elderly treated within the institutional care is three times higher when compared to the same number of individuals from general population and female patients need twice as many drugs as the male ones. In order to achieve maximum elimination of side effects of pharmacotherapy we should apply following *principles of treating patients of advanced age* [61]:

A. Minimum drugs
B. The shortest possible period of drug administration
C. Use lower but effective dosages
D. Consider drug interactions
E. Non-pharmacological treatment whenever applicable.

Higher occurrence of undesired drug effects and higher susceptibility to them in the elderly is to a certain extent caused by automatic prescribing of drugs in this group of patients without any continuous analysis of the clinical status which should be performed by the physician who is responsible for the patient.

Main role in achieving desired effect of the drug is played by pharmaco-kinetics and pharmaco-dynamics of drugs. Both these processes can be modified in advanced age by physiological changes caused by organ ageing and at the same time multi-morbidity. The drug can be effective only if it arrives in proper place sufficiently concentrated.

Phamaco-kinetics is based prevailingly on the changes of bio-chemical and physiological functions of an organism [54]. It deals with changes of the drug concentration in the course of time in various compartments of an organism from the moment of an input (drug administration) up to the receptors. Its potential changes in advanced age in the course of several stages are analyzed in table 2.

Table 2. Pharmaco-kinetical changes in advanced age

Pharmaco-kinetical changes in advanced age
1. Absorption of drugs
2. Distribution of drugs
3. Bio-transformation of drugs
4. Elimination of drugs

Pharmaco-kinetical changes correlate with changes of body and elimination organ composition. Decrease of lean body mass and proportion of total somatic water (including extra-cellular) and on the other hand increase of proportion of total somatic adipose tissue lead to changes in drug distribution depending on their solubility and protein bonds. Percentage of somatic fat increases up to the age of 85 and decreases afterwards, therefore liposoluble substances have prolonged effect. The volume of distribution of drugs is also affected. Since older adults have a decrease in total body water and a relative increase in body fat, water-soluble drugs become more concentrated and fat-soluble drugs have longer half-lives.

Distribution of drugs depends on the body composition as mentioned, bonds to plasmatic proteins and blood flow trough tissues. Poorly nourished or frail elderly persons may have a low serum albumin. A cardiac output in advanced age decreases, peripheral vessel resistance grows, liver gets smaller and blood flow trough liver and kidneys decreases. Bigger part of the cardiac output in comparison to the younger ones flows through the brains, heart and skeleton muscles. This also plays a role in the drug distribution.

Hepatic metabolism also may decline with age. Oxidative reactions, so-called phase 1 reactions, become impaired with normal ageing, whereas phase 2 reactions (acetylation, sulphatation, glucuronidization) are relatively spared. These enzyme changes are (especially in the elderly) intra-individually very variable. The decrease of drug metabolism as a consequence of the said CYP 450 can be 20 – 40 per cent (teophyllin, some beta-blockers, calcium channel blockers, antidepressants). Moreover renal functions in advanced age decrease with various velocity up to 30 – 50 per cent of original level which reduces renal elimination of numerous drugs. Exceptionally however renal functions can be completely preserved up to the advanced age. Renal clearence of many drugs is decreased in old age and well correlates with reduced glomerular filtration.

The overall impact of these pharmacokinetic changes is that the half-life, which is proportional to the volume of distribution divided by drug clearance, increases for many lipophilic drugs.

Pharmaco-dynamics is considered a basis of pharmacology [54]. Drug effects are based first of all on specific interactions of substances of biological systems – *receptor mechanisms*. A receptor is a mediator for the substance which interacts with it and thus brings specific response. Physiological changes and a loss of homeostatic flexibility lead to increased sensitivity to undesired drug effects - e.g. hypotension after psychopharmacs and haemorrhage after anticoagulant agents.

Significant changes in numerous drug effects can be found in most people of advanced age. The range of applicable drugs changes in the old age and tends gradually to polypharmacotherapy. Multi-morbidity is a typical feature as well as nutritional problems and increasing risk of non-compliance. These facts when combined with pharmaco-kinetical and pharmaco-dynamical changes may lead up to serious undesired side effects and drug interactions. Increasing age brings generally increased iterindividual variability of dosages needcd for achieving the therapeutical effect. Pharmacotherapy in geriatric patients can be not only significantly curative but also dangerously toxic.

Chapter 9

Problems and Complications of Polypharmacy

Occurrence of *undesired drug effects* is generally 3 – 5 times higher in advanced age when compared to preceding age categories [9]. Higher consumption of drugs brings along higher risks. Side effects occur in 2 per cent of the elderly using less than 3 drugs at a time during a year. This percentage grows up to 17 in those who use 10 drugs. Combination of more drugs is preferred recently more and more frequently to mono-therapy. Except for expected and beneficial effect of synergism it can bring also adverse side effects. Number of new drugs especially in psychiatry and neurology grows dramatically during last decades. The most frequently prescribed drugs today are anxiolytics and antidepressants. They are often required also by the elderly and their usage grows also in internal medicine, geriatrics and other non-psychiatric medical branches. One third of the undesired drug effect is predictable and mere reduction of a dosage can eliminate two thirds of them. There is justified question whether standard dosages recommended to general application are not too high for the elderly. Moreover these undesired effects are often atypical in the elderly (such as confusion, depression, parkinsonism, falls, incontinence etc.). It was proved that long-term administration of benzodiazepins in combination therapy together with four and more other drugs often leads to falls [21,79]. The risk of fall is 2.5 times higher with benzodiazepin alone but 28 times higher with drug combinations.

These undesired effects are often wrongly diagnosed which leads to prescription and administration of further drugs – it is a so called *prescriptive cascade.* Correct medication (both with prescription drugs and commercially available medicaments) is based on the right indication appropriate dosage and forms adapted to intellectual potential and somatic skills of a patient, elimination of predictable undesired effects and drug interactions and minimisation of their impacts on patient, consideration of optimum period of drug administration and consistent monitoring of permanent administration connected with continuous evaluation of compliance [54].

The older people are more sensitive to drug effects and clinical consequences of the undesired effects lead to hospitalisation in up to 10 per cent of cases. Although the proportion of advanced age population in industrial countries is about 1/5 – 1/8 their consumption of drugs is up to 1/3 of the whole. Moreover these patients take up to 2 commercially available drugs. Problems with drug administration in advanced age are common especially if the dosage scheme is complicated. The best of all is to establish the simplest possible dosage regimen with intervals once or twice daily. Non-compliance occurs in 25 – 50 per cent of older patients taking drugs regularly.

When prescribing a drug the physician should ask:

- Which drug is the most convenient one regarding multi-morbidity and predictable drug interactions?
- What is the optimum dosage?
- Is a drug indication definite and undoubtful?

Chapter 10

MULTI-MORBIDITY IN OLD AGE AND ITS RELATIONS

The interaction between old age and illness causes specific changes of diseases in senium [9,79,86].

Particularities of illness in old age include:

- Multi-morbidity – parallel occurrence of more illnesses in one person with or without causality relationship
- Mutual causality of social and health situation – each of the changes of the health state in old age influences their social status and vice versa
- Among the specialities of clinical picture of illnesses in old age we can list:

1. *microsymptomathology* – minimal symptoms of diseases (the iceberg phenomenon)
2. *mono- or oligosyptomatology* – sporadic symptoms from those, which occur usually in middle or young age
3. *distant signs* – to the forefront of clinical picture there are symptoms, which belong to the difficulties of other organ than the basic one ("the innocent organ complains, not the sick one")
4. *tendency to chronicity* – even in the diseases which are in younger and middle age acute, moreover in old age there is higher risk of death
5. *tendency to complications* - either of type of "chain reaction" or it is the complication, which does not have the direct relation ("crowd-out effect")

6. *atypical picture* of the diseases – *„For the diseases in the old age it is typical that their running is atypical"*

The proper symptomathology of the basic disease is usually inconspicuous. In the clinical picture manifestation of non-specific and universal symptoms dominates. These are the results of the *secondary brain decompensation.* Among those the universal *neurologic and psychiatric symptomathology* conditioned on hypo-perfusion (hypoxia) of the brain (TIA, delirium etc.) belong. The senior's brain is usually affected with the degenerative or vascular changes and reacts usually as the first organ.

Among the causes of the morbidity in old age the forward position [107] is being taken by the diseases of the cardiovascular system conditioned with atherosclerosis like CHD (coronary heart disease), MI (myocardial infarckt), angina pectoris, stroke, transient ischemic attack, ischemic disease of the lower limbs (atherosclerosis - AS is present in 90% of the people above 75 years.). In old age we find common: the diseases of the locomotive system, sense organs, tumours, accidental injuries, the diseases of the respiratory tract, gastrointestinal tract (biliary problems etc.) and urogenital tract (the prostate in men, gynecological in women). Diabetes, mental and neurological disorders are common [8,102]. Their coincidental and usually independent occurrence is typical for the senior's multi-morbidity. After the age of 60 there is continuous increase mainly of the cardiovascular diseases as CHD, stroke, hypertension [31,78]. Similarly with the age prevalence of diabetes rises [101].

For the quality of the senior's life crucial matter is not the presence of the disease itself (or more diseases) but the grade of the disability, it means functional disturbance, into which it is proceeding. The full self-sufficiency can be untouched even when there are more diseases present together.

The inclination of the seniors to the diseases is higher [58] and the balance of the organ homeostasis is very frail (eg. homeostenosis). Similarly it is the case of "primary" mental disorders (dementia, depression, delirium) or in the geriatric social syndromes (neglect sy, elder abuse, geriatric maladaptation sy). The stressor is usually in psychosocial sphere and its clinical manifestation appears most often in cardiovascular area (heart failure, MI, stroke) or in impaired immunity (pneumonia).

As it was mentioned, the diseases and the morbid conditions in old age are marked by many extraordinarities. The diseases in old age have the tendency to cumulate and potentiate each other. In the geriatric medicine multidimensionality is typical. It is needed to comprehend the sick person in old age as the bio-psycho-social unit in more holistic way than in younger age from the viewpoint of etiopatogenesis of the disease and also in the case of everyday clinical practice.

The quoted problems from the somatic, psychic and social areas which are in the mutual interaction are hardly treatable, they are chronic with the progression of the condition and they have relatively unfavourable prognosis. They bring a lot of hardly solvable situations and problems to the ill and the surroundings. By the „old old“ people ($\geq$ 80 years) the diseases proceed in the way, which differ from the progress of the diseases in middle age and they need the different approach which can improve the health condition or at least maintain the self-sufficiency and they accent the comeback home.

The most of the biological functions achieve the top before the 30th year of the life. Some of them slightly decrease afterwards linearly. For the everyday activity this decrease has not any practical importance, but can be relevant in the time of bigger stress or in the load. The physiological processes which are decreasing as the age grows are: blood flow through the kidneys, the clearance of the creatinin, the maximum heart rate and pulse volume in stress, glucose tolerance, vital capacity of the lungs, body weight, cell immunity. On the contrary the total lung capacity and the liver function do not change with increasing age, the production of the ADH is even growing.

Many of mentioned declines, which were thought as natural consequence of the ageing, are significantly influenced by the life style, behaviour, diet and environment in which the senior has been living. The most important physiological change in old age is the predisposition to the higher occurrence of severe diseases. The respiratory functions of a 70 year old healthy man are the 50% of the 30 years old man. The renal function usually goes down in 70 years by 50% and more. This decline in physiological reserve capacity does not influence the everyday life but it can influence the ability to recover from the severe disease (grave infection, life threatening internal diseases, operations, injuries etc.)

Some of the physiological changes can simulate a disease even if they are just a usual component of the ageing. Diabetes mellitus can appear and disappear in the old age. The ability of the insulin to stimulate the take up of the glucose declines with the age and is usually manifested as postprandial hyperglycaemia with normal fasting level of insulin and glucose. In the stress situations diabetes can be detected in seniors, but it can disappear when the situation gets normal. This loss of the physiological reserves contributes to the rising prevalence of diabetes with the rising age.

The age conditioned changes, which make the old age people more vulnerable in their everyday life, are usually mild. In the elderly there is an onset of hypo- or hyperthermia easier during the exposition to extreme surrounding influences, because there are a lot of changes in the coordination of the lead of the thermoregulation also in the neurological area. The loss of neurotransmitters in brain stem can cause typical senile walk, as well as it predisposes genetically determined individuals for e.g. to the progress of the Parkinson‘s disease. Some of the age conditioned changes cause the specific consequences. The menopausis is the physiological process connected with normal ageing but it leads to the symptoms, which predispose the organism to the loss of the bone mass and atherosclerosis.

Apart from clinically obvious forms of the diseases in the elderly the sub-clinical form is common as well. Among 6 000 individuals above 65 years which were in the Cardiovascular Health Study [33] 31% of them had clinically apparent cardiovascular disease, another 37% had sub-clinical form of the disease which was found by non-invasive methods.

The half of the people above 65 years have two or more diseases and these can mean an added risk of unfavourable consequences like mortality. In some of the seniors the cognitive disturbance can imitate symptoms of a severe disease. The therapy of one disease can act in an undesirable way on the other place – such as e.g. use of aspirin as the prevention of the ictus in the individual with the anamnesis of the gastroduodenal ulcer. The risk leading to disability or dependence on the help is getting higher with the number of co-morbidities. Certain couplets of the diseases can increase the risk of disability synergistically. The arthrosis and the diseases of the heart co-exist in 1/5 of the elderly, even though the risks of progress of disability are 3- or 4-times higher with one of them alone, the risk of both together is 14-times higher [21].

At the end the severe and common consequence of the chronic disease in old age is physical disability, defined as the presence of difficulties or dependence on the others when doing common everyday activities, from the basic self-service (the toilet and washing up) to the tasks needed for leading the independent life (shopping, preparing food, paying the bills etc.).

On the onset and the progress of the critical conditions in old age following factors can significantly participate: *the poor mobility, loneliness, bad eating habits, insufficient hydration, mental deterioration, disturbance of the sight and hearing*. The mentioned ill individuals have, as it is with multi-morbidity in old age common, an atypical picture, or they can be without symptoms or the problems are seemingly moved to the other organ area. The important role is played also often by rich pharmacotherapy in old age, which can itself cause different organ symptoms (also by the mutual interactions).

The management of the critical ill persons in old age will demand very active approach from the clinical doctors (incl. intensivists) and sometimes also usage of more invasive procedures in the diagnostics and therapy, which can act unfavourably in some of the cases and sometimes also iatrogenically.

Chapter 11

ORGAN SYSTEMS IN OLD AGE AND THEIR SPECIFICS

I consider it necessary at least through this short notice to point out organ specificities, which can become the reason to accept the patient to ICU. The following paragraphs summarize the examples of more severe physiological changes observed in the older age according to the organ systems.

THE COMPOSITION OF THE ORGANISM AND HOMEOSTASIS

The changes in the body composition include the decrease of lean body mass (primarily the consequence of the loss of the muscles) connected with the proportional increase of the body fat [56,81,118]. These basic changes are important determinants of the physiological functions and therapeutical intervention in the elderly. For example the reduced muscle tissue is responsible to a certain extent for the decline of consumption of oxygen during the exercise ($VO_{2max.}$) detectable with the growing age. Moreover the elevation of the body fat enlarges the distributional volume of lipophile drugs and thus prolongs their pharmacological action. The changes in the body composition in seniors are probably caused both by the process of ageing and those external factors like physical inactivity and changed way of alimentation. The age changes include homeostatic control of disturbed baro-reflex sensitivity, which alone predispose to orthostatic hypotension a worse thermoregulation, which elevates the tendency to hypothermia and stroke.

THE CARDIOVASCULAR SYSTEM

Many studies were conducted for the evaluation of the functional changes of cardiovascular system in old age [15]. An example of properly documented observation is a model of fulfilling of the left ventricle which changes with age. In old age the early diastolic volume is smaller a so are the atrial contractions elevated, so that the adequate volume of the left ventricle is maintained [63]. With age the contents of the connective tissue elevates as well as the presence of ventricular hypertrophy. The consequence of the elevated left-ventricular rigidity can develop the symptoms of the lung congestion in seniors (murmurs, dyspnoe on exertion) even without any systolic dysfunction. In seniors the *diastolic dysfunction* has principal relevance [3]. The augmentation of the contraction force by the medicament like digoxin does not act for the desired purpose and can be harmful for the patient [115]. The slight enhancement of the therapy by diuretics and strict control of co-existing hypertension is the most useful therapeutical modality in such patients. During an intensive loading the heart rate elevates less than in the younger. This age conditioned change, is usually assigned to the weakening beta-adrenergic influence of the heart rate during the load [16]. Even though the hypertension is not possible to consider physiological manifestation of ageing, its incidence increases with age and higher blood pressure accelerates the ageing process and the connected organ changes. More than a half of the seniors are hypertonics and they can gain in a various extent from proper modifications of the life style, or pharmacotherapy. The arterial rigidity increases with the age [14], too which is of the multi-factorial origin [67]. Factors participating in this process are hypertension, elevated deposition of collagen into the arterial walls, calcifications and proceeding atherosclerosis. On the other side, the old age modifies the clinical picture, the therapeutical procedure and prognosis in older hypertonics. The therapy of hypertension of seniors leads to a decline in the number of brain strokes and in minor extent also in decrease of the cardiovascular attacks.

THE RESPIRATORY SYSTEM

The most typical change of the old age thorax is the rigidity [78]. The lung functions lower with the rising age [71]. During the ageing the elastic component in lungs becomes smaller and the loss of alveoli tightly connected by the elastic fibres happens. The reduced elasticity of the lungs contributes to age conditioned elevation of functional residual capacity (calm breath out) and residual volume [23]. The loss of the elasticity leads early to collapse of the peripheral respiratory ways during the intensive breath out, and it can partially lead to age conditioned reduction of the maximum vital capacity (intensive breath out after the maximum inspiration) and of the volume of intensive breath out volume during one second (forced expiratory volume in 1 sec. - FEV_1). Moreover the reduced elasticity progressively elevates the closing pressure in the breath ways in such an extent, that in some of the older individuals this closure can occur also during normal breathing.

The loss of the maximum breath capacity is by 40% [109]. On the level of the alveoli the exchange of the oxygen and carbonic oxide is reduced approximately by 50% in the age range 30 to 65 years [78]. Even though these changes are not observable in the rest, the older individuals feel tired or the shortage of the breath with higher labour (exercise or severe disease). The lung reflexes like cough (ciliary function) get lower with the increasing age and so predispose the elderly to accumulate the secretions and to the development of the aspiratory pneumonia [116].

The arterial oxygen pressure is reduced with the age in relatively wide range as the result of imbalance of the ventilation and perfusion [71]. The lowered ventilation reaction to hypoxia and hypercapnia is demonstratable in older people and it is considered to be the decline of the function of chemoreceptors. All these changes do not lead to fundamental changes in rest oxygen saturation but decrease the arterial PO_2. The arterial PO_2 of a lot of individuals above 80 years old is about 70 – 75 mmHg. These changes of blood gases play the minimal role in rest conditions, but dramatically influence the survival during the severe respiratory diseases [88].

THE GASTRO-INTESTINAL TRACT

During the process of ageing the function of the GIT (gastrointestinal tract) is changed relatively little in comparison to the other organ systems [62]. Probably it is thanks to elevation of the secretion of GIT hormones and so the relative structural surplus of this system. In old age the slight reduction of the motility, secretion of the digestive juices and absorption of the food take place [30]. A lot of specific dyspeptic problems have more or less functional character and it is more in relation to the multi-morbidity of the individual proper. Nevertheless the GIT is in old age more vulnerable in terms of the diseases and their incidence grows with the age [118]. Moreover the symptoms of many GIT diseases in old age have complex character, are discrete and there can be difficulties with the diagnostics. In older age also the differential diagnostics of various problems is very important and difficult, like e.g. breast pain (angina pectoris versus gastroesophageal reflux – up to 30%) or symptoms in the area of the abdomen at all [40,108]. With increasing atherosclerotic affection of the abdominal vessels also the occurrence of various angiodysplasias grows, bleeding lesions of GIT, complications of vascular ischemia (ischemic colitis, vascular ileus) take place, which do not occur in the younger ones.

The Uropoetic System

The gradual decrease of the renal function becomes after 40th year by about 1ml/min/year [24]. The glomerular filtration evaluated by the clearance of creatinin can decrease even by 1/3 of original value [7]. However this decrease does not come in 1/3 of people, so it can not be attributed to the involution. Apart from the reduction of the function of glomeruli, the renal perfusion, tubular resorption (eg. glucose, sodium), concentrational and dilutional ability reduces with the age too [84]. The serum creatinin thanks to the reduction of the whole muscle mass can have the smaller outcome value than in the younger ones. The renal insufficiency [51] – also chronic - has increasing tendency with increasing age thanks to the damage of the glomeruli (e.g. diabetic nephropathy) and ischemic nephropathy (hypertension, atherosclerosis).

The *internal homeostasis* is usually a sign of all of the extracellular fluid composed by interstitial and intravasal fluid (i.e. means blood plasma). It makes the dynamic system maintaining permanent homeostasis in the organism [7]. The higher age is not connected in healthy seniors with changes of electrolytes or acid-base homeostasis. The changes of main serum ions: sodium, potassium, chlorides, are not present. The carbonic oxide is not changed either. Just very slight decrease takes place with pH [6]. Urea in contrast to creatinin has the increasing tendency with the age (correlation with the progression of sclerosis of glomeruli). In the stress like the disease, the urea and creatinin increase in the serum in seniors. With the disease in old age the occurrence of ion disturbance and acid-base homeostasis increases, because the reins in senium have impaired ability to react effectively to aberrations of electrolytes and acid-base homeostasis [51]. The occurrence of the complications resulting from the disability to maintain stabile ion homeostasis increases with the presence of intermittent diseases and mainly in critical states. In concordance with the decrease of the glomerular function also the tubular dysfunction takes place (disturbance of reuptake of glucose and sodium). The renal ATP-asis is in decrease, also the reuptake of sodium by tubules decreases, losses of sodium and water increase, the exchange of sodium-hydrogen and sodium-phosphate decreases in comparison with the younger ones. Acid-base (AB) homeostasis is maintained also in old age in the narrow range of pH 7.35 – 7.45.

The age will limit the ability of right reaction to stress by compensatory mechanisms of lungs and reins [23]. E.g. the ability of the lungs to react by hyperventilation to an acute metabolic acidosis is weakened and leads to further decrease of the pH. The ageing reins also react more slowly to the loading of acids and the pH of the blood recovers more slowly. Many of the diseases which occur in the higher age (like heart failure, anaemia, sepsis, diabetes mellitus, renal and lung diseases) can excessively burden the regulatory systems and can contribute to the progression of acid-base disturbances. Similarly numerous medicaments used in senium (NSAD, diuretics, laxatives) can contribute to AB dysbalances. The combination of slightly impaired homeostasis and polymorbidity together with polypharmacotherapy in older age lead to the fact, that impairment of the acid-base homeostasis are common. In spite of the increase in the excretion of the antidiuretic hormone, the reactivity of the rein to it decreases with the age, which leads into reduced concentration ability of the reins after water deprivation. Moreover in the elderly the feeling of thirst is reduced and also the drinking regime with lack of water. Impaired concentration ability of the reins and reduced feeling of thirst in old age can significantly enlarge the risk of dehydration during any severe disease.

THE ENDOCRINE SYSTEM

The extraordinary attention is paid to the changes of the glucose metabolism connected with the ageing. Glucose tolerance decreases with the age. In the healthy seniors the plasma glucose measured 2 hours after the loading of the glucose in oral glucose toleration test is increasing from the age of 50 years on by about 0,33 – 0,72 mmol/l (6.6-14.4mg%) per decade; whilst fasting glycemia elevates only by 0,05 – 0,06 mmol/l (1-1.2mg%) per decade [87]. This impairment of the glucose toleration in advanced age is independent on obesity and physical inactivity, which are common in the process of ageing and can themselves contribute to the progression of the glucose intolerance. The primary cause of the impairment of glucose intolerance during the ageing is the insulin resistance in the peripheral tissue, especially in the muscles. The numerous studies [101] documented, that the bond of insulin on the cell receptors change does not occur with the age, so the cause of impaired glucose intolerance which is age conditioned is the post-receptor abnormality of insulin action (i.e. intracellular defect).

Even though the insulin secretion can be impaired in old age, the levels of circulating insulin are not decreased probably because thanks to age conditioned decrease of insulin clearance. The impaired glucose toleration during old age is not really the same as the glycemia in diabetics. Nevertheless according to the theory of ageing which puts the accent on the binding the glucose on the proteins there could also be the long term elevations of the glycemia influence the process of physiological deterioration or the diseases typically occurring in old age. From this point of view the fasting glycemia and glycosylated haemoglobin embody the high grade of correlation in non-diabetics of higher age in the wider sense of the word. Some of the epidemiological studies show, that elevations of the glycemia also in non-diabetics can accent the process of cardiovascular diseases. The optimum fasting glycemia of diabetics should be according to Sinclair [101] in range less than 7 mmol/l (HbA_{1C} 4.2-5%), but it should not be above 9-10 mmol/l (HbA_{1C} > 5% < 6%) even in very old, disabled diabetics. Even those disabled older diabetics should not be in danger of acute hypoglycemia. DM concern in the 7th decade up to 20% of people and further 20% suffer from impaired glucose toleration [102]. It is the most important metabolic disease of the older age. In seniors it is mainly DM 2nd type (among all the diabetics above 70 years up to 95%).

Another endocrine variable of potential significance during ageing is the growth hormone (GH) and insulin-like growth factor1 (IGF-1). The pituitary secretion of the growth hormone is decreasing with the age. Much of the anabolic effects of GH [64] is mediated by IGF-1, which is produced in the liver and other tissues on GH impulse. Similarly as the GH [113] decreases in old age, also the secretion of IGF-1 decreases. The changes of the body composition in senium (it means the reduction of muscles and elevation of tissue fat) are very close to the changes occurring in the younger individuals with the deficiency of the growth hormone [25]. These findings lead to the hypothesis, that typical changes in old age are conditioned by reduction of the secretion of the growth hormone [76].

During ageing there can be beginning of atrophy, fibrosis, an increase of coloid nodes and lymphocyte infiltration in the thyroid gland observed [103]. In senium cases of thyreopathy will be found in up to one tenth of the individuals, more in women. Often it will be only in the laboratory results without any clinical symptoms, it means subclinical hypothyreosis and hypothyreosis with the deviation of TSH without the change in thyroxine (T_4). The consideration whether to begin the therapy of subclinical hypo- or hyperthyreosis belongs to the very controversial questions with the fact, that the crucial will be the whole clinical picture and the grade of possible influenceable symptoms from the hypo- or hyperfunction of the thyroid gland. The prevalence of hypothyreosis significantly rises in old age. Its clinical symptomathology is much less obvious than in younger individuals. The secretion of the thyroxine is reduced by 30% in comparison to the young adults, whilst plasma level of thyroxine remains unchanged. This decrease of secretion of T_4 is considered physiological compensation of reduced use in the tissue and not the manifestation of the primary thyreopathy. The reduced utilisation of T_4 correlates with reduced active muscle tissue of the organism. With the age also the level of TSH slightly increases which can probably explain the higher occurrence of Hashimoto thyreoiditis in senium. The autoimmune thyreoditis occurs up to 1-2% of the older population, mainly of women. The compensatory process in old age is also slight decrease of deiodation in periphery to T_3.

The ovaria show the dramatic decrease of secretion of estrogen and progesteron in old age and also fibrosis and scars. Menopausis is the most important age conditioned endocrine syndrome. Menopausis occurs in average in the age of about 50 years with concomitant rush, the loss of bone mass and estrogen-sensitive tissue is accented. Andropausis in men with decreasing level of testosteron begins after 50th year (without the influence on potency). The sexual functions are relatively well protected, even if the increase of refractory period and prolonging of the time needed to sexual excitement and loss of tissue turgor. Menopause is the most important age-related endocrine syndrome.

The Immune System

The decrease of immune functions predisposes the older people to higher occurrence of the infectious diseases and malignancies [46,75]. Typical for the higher age is the reduction of the cell immunity with reduction of T lymphocytes in the answer on the mitogenic stimulation. Impaired proliferation of T-cells in old age can be responsible for defective intracellular transduction of mitogenic signals [18]. Moreover the synthesis of interleukine-2 (IL-2) and IL-2 receptor expression, which are necessary for the proliferation of T-cells, are both reduced in the later old age. The involution of the thymus and loss of its hormones play an essential role in the decrease of the function of T-cells in senium. Age conditioned changes of humoral immunity conclude the elevated production of the auto-antibodies and decrease in antibody reaction to alien stimulation. These changes reflect age conditioned deviation of the functions of T- and B-cells.

The Musculosceletal System

The bone mass and the density is reduced with the age after 20 years achieved [50]. In women until the menopausis this loss is up to 1% per year, but then it may increase to 2 or 3%. After 5 -10 years after the menopausis the bone loss is back to 1% per year, but it can accelerate again in about 80th year of age. The men have primarily larger bone mass than women, the loss is also 1% per year, but the clinical effect is not visible until the late senium. The tendons and ligaments become less elastic in old age, which can lead to higher incidence of the rupture (Achilles tendon). The cartilage of the ribs and the spine are less elastic and more calcificated. The muscles in 70 years are reduced by 25% in men and women. In 80 years the muscle size and force in the individuals with prevailingly sedentary lifestyle are reduced by 30%-40% [32].

The Visual Disturbances

They occur in 1 of 6 people in the age of 75-84 years and in every fourth individual above 85 years [21]. 1% of people above 65 are disabled by almost loss of the vision. Among the important causes of the impairment of the sight in old age the macular degeneration, cataract, diabetic retinopathy and glaucoma belong. In old age also the impairments of the accommodation of the lens appear more frequently, which can be corrected by the glasses or contact lenses. The loss of the sight is connected with complete loss of the independence, reduction of the physical activity and depression. The risk of falls and injuries increases as well.

THE HEARING IMPAIRMENTS

Clinically important hearing impairment occurs in 1/3 of the individuals above 65 years and in ½ of people above 75 years [79]. The most common impairment is presbyacusis with the loss of high-frequency tones, which can be improved by use of the hearing aids.

Chapter 12

DEHYDRATION – WATER, NATRIUM AND POTASSIUM DISTURBANCES IN THE ELDERLY

With age, total body water decreases [6] because of an increase in fat and a decrease in lean body mass (from about 60% of body weight in healthy young adults to about 45% of body weight in the elderly). Ageing is associated with impaired water conservation and sodium balance-factors that determine extracellular fluid (ECF) volume and tonicity [12]. Thirst and the secretion of antidiuretic hormone (ADH) control water balance. The elderly have delayed and less intense thirst response than younger persons. The older body tends to secrete ADH despite decreased blood tonicity (the syndrome of inappropriate ADH secretion [SIADH], especially in a person with chronic cardiac, hepatic, or renal disease. The ability to concentrate urine decreases with age in part because of tubular senescence.

DEHYDRATION

It is a very important problem in the elderly and it is usually a matter of everyday clinical practice. Common clinical attribute is the thirst, tachycardia, orthostatic hypotension, reduced skin turgor, dry mucous membranes and decrease of diuresis; also central venous pressure will be reduced. Very useful for the evaluation of the fluid movement at ICU will be regular weight measurment. There is a risk of its quick development in the elderly because the protective mechanisms are missing (the feeling of the thirst) and the balance is very frail [53]. Multi-morbidity is often connected with diuretics therapy [1]. In the laboratory findings there will be common growth of haemoglobine, haematocrite and total protein. Natrium and osmolality will be different [90]. In principle dehydration can be of three types [43]:

Isotonic Dehydration

Typical is steady decrease of natrium and water (in serum normal!). The cause could be most frequently insufficiently substituted losses of natrium and water by diuretics therapy, polyuric phase of chronic renal insufficiency, diarrhoea, constipation etc. It is necessary to replenish the volume of fluids - at ICU usually with infusions (0.9% sodium chloride).

Hypotonic Dehydration

Loss of sodium overhangs loss of water. It can be the consequence of diuretic therapy or other losses of natrium, when replaced predominantly with free water. This *dilutional hyponatremia* we discover often in persons with heart or renal failure, liver cirrhosis, if is present secondary hyperaldosteronism, ADH secretion increases and long/term are used diuretics. We assess hyponatremia and hypoosmolality with risk of transfer free water into the cells. Brain edema threatens with all possible complications (cramps, consciousness disturbances, death). In critically ill patients it is necessary to apply a no-delay infusion therapy (0.9% sodium chloride). In chronical states it is suitable to carry out restriction of fluids, concomitant diuretics administration with running metabolic control. Dialysis is indicated in cases of renal insufficiency.

Hypertonic Dehydration

We can characterize it in comparison to the previous ones with elevated serum natrium and osmolality as the result of the deficit of free water. The cause in the elderly will be mostly osmotically affecting diuretics, hyperglycemia, bad potable regimen exaggerated with lost feeling of thirst. There are fully indicated solutions of 5% dextrose.

HYPERHYDRATION

It is totally elevated volume of ECF, which will be in the elderly similarly important as dehydration. Etiologically the cause will be usually conditions connected with retention of fluids as heart and renal failure and others (especially secondary hyperaldosteronism). Clinically the state will be represented with increased weight, that will cause swellings and exudates (ascites, fluidothorax etc) as the sign of circulatory failure. In laboratory finding there will be a decrease of haemoglobin present, haematocrit and total protein, that will be uniform in all conditions. Natrium and osmolality will be different according to the kind of hyperhydration. Hyperhydration may be of three types as well as the dehydratation:

Isotonic Hyperhydration

It is caused by elevated natrium and osmolality with swellings – often with heart congestion. Specific weight of urine is normal. In the therapy it is necessary to focus on the evoking disease and to treat it more comprehensively (including modification of diuretic doses).

Hypotonic Hyperhydration

This situation threatens mainly in critical conditions as the result of excessive administration of free water. Sodium, osmolality (in serum) and specific weight of urine are reduced. Natrium must not be administred for the risk of further retention of water. Treatment is the arrangement of the relations (in case of need also by diuretics) and mainly good adjustment of infusion solutions with sufficient contents of solutes.

Hypertonic Hyperhydration

This derangement may lead to exceeded intake of water with excessive natrium supply (iatrogenically as consequence of inappropriate infusion solution treatment). Natrium, osmolality and specific weight of urine are elevated. It is inevitable to stop natrium influx immediately.

Natrium

It is a cardinal caution unavoidable for the maintenance of stable osmotic pressure and regulation of the volume ECF [105,110]. Its normal serum level is 135-145 mmol/l and excretion in urine 70-270 mmol/24 h. Its oscilations can go with both dehydration and hyperhydration (see above).

Hyponatremia

Sodium in serum < 135 mmol/l may accompany both situations (both dehydratation and hyperhydration) and was discussed above. It can affect nearly ¼ long-term ill seniors. Hyponatremia consequently can be hypo-, iso- and hypervolemic. Hyponatremia is usual condition connected with massive swellings accompanied moreover with hypoproteinemia (dilutional hyponatremia).

Symptomatic hyponatremia is the one that develops during 48 hours. Cephalea, seizures, coma eventually death according to developing brain's oedema.

In contrast to the previous ones there will be *asymptomatic hyponatremia* accompanying chronical states as described above and therapeutic approach will be more conservative.

Hypernatremia

Natrium in serum > 150 mmol/l may accompany both dehydratation and hyperhydration. In patients at ICU it is assessed at admission time nearly in 9% and during the stay at ICU in further 6%. Hypertonic dehydration will be again often in seniors due to loss of the thirst feeling.

Potassium

Potassium in serum varies in range 3,8-5,1 mmol/l (1). Urine scrap by its 90% excretion through urine should be 25-125 mmol/24 hours. It represents one of the most essential intracellular caution, where the bulk of it is situated. Extracellularly it is located only in 2% and that is why it is very difficult to deduce its real stores from its serum value in ECF. Excretion of potassium to urine/24 h. predicates better about its movement ion body. In seniors we can often encounter both hypo- and hyperkalemia thanks to present multi-morbidity and frequently used treatment with diuretics. In general alterations of serum potassium are the most dangerous, they develop rapidly. Hypokalemia is always the sign of intracellular potassium deficit. Hyperkalemia may accompany both normal and elevated value in cells.

Hypokalemia

It is usually defined as serum level < 3,5 mmol/l and is actually assessed at 20% hospitalized seniors in ICU. This fact probably in majority of them does not signalize potassium depletion. The cause of hypokalemia apart from diuretic therapy can be diarrhoe, intestinal atonia, vomiting, polyuric phase of chronic renal failure [57] and secondary hyperaldosteronism as accompanying manifestation of the diseases with fluid retention (heart failure, liver cirrhosis and the like).

In clinical picture GI disorders swallowing, sinking of intestinal motility, constipation, parestesia, cardiomuscullary symptoms with hypotension and overall muscle weakness and threat of heart dysrhytmia dominate. Diagnostically in ECG depression ST segment; decrease till inversion T wave; visualisation of U wave, sometimes fusion T and U waves appear. Patients with hypokalemia are two-fold prone to development of ventricular fibrilation. Digitalis toxicity grows together with risk of dysrhytmia and also in normal digoxin value in serum is risky. Persons with K < 3,0 suffer from constipation and < 2,5 mmol/l paralytic ileus.

Treatment by K < 3,0 mmol/l consists in oral administration of potassium. More aggressive procedure instead is at ICU in persons with hypertension, case-history of heart failure and enhanced risk of cardiac dysrhytmia or stroke in anamnesis. At ICU potassium must be administred solely by injector or infusion pump with velocity 10-20 ml/h. in 500 ml solution, but maximally KCl 100-200 mmol/24h.

Hyperkalemia

It appears usually in renal insufficiency, both chronic and acute, (with metabolic acidosis), hyperglycemia connected with ketoacidosis or developed iatrogenically (potassium saving diuretics, beta-blockers, ACE-I, AT II blockers, NSA etc.). Hyperkalemia with metabolic acidosis develops by mechanism of enhanced shift K^+ out of the cells and H^+ into these spaces, that bounds to phosphate.

In clinical status symptomatology of cardiovascular system dominate. Patients are hypotensive and prone to the development of dysrhytmia (bradycardiac form). On ECG occurrs enlargement QRS complex, shortening and depression ST segment, and formation tall, narrow T waves . The predisposition to ventricular fibrilation is higher.

In treatment it is suitable to use infusion 20-40% dextrose 500 ml with insulin (40-80 j. to central vein; pertinently at least 10% dextrose in peripheral vein. With dysrhytmias we can administer also 20 ml calcium gluconicum or $CaCl_2$ slowly iv. or in iv. infusion. At values 6,2-6,5 mmol/l (according to pH) dialysis is fully indicated.

Chapter 13

DELIRIUM

Delirium is an acute, fluctuating alteration in level of consciousness and attention. It is a common occurrence, particularly in hospitalized elderly patients [10,43]. It occurs in 20% to 30% of elderly patients admitted with an acute medical diagnosis. Risk factors for incident delirium in hospitalized elderly patients include baseline dementia, severe underlying illness, sensory impairment, and dehydration [12,29]. Since its manifestations can be variable, it is often overlooked. Delirium is associated with increased morbidity and care expenses. It may be precipitated by processes of hospital care, including immobilization of the patient, use of an indwelling bladder catheter, use of physical restraints, dehydration, malnutrition, iatrogenic complications, and psychosocial factors [97,111]. Delirium prolongs hospital length of stay, increases costs of care, and increases the risk of nursing home placement or death. It belongs to the most frequent and most serious mental disorders occurring in advanced age.

EPIDEMIOLOGY AND ETIOLOGY

Delirium is very common among the elderly. Of general medical patients ≥ 70 years admitted to the hospital, 10 to 20% are delirious at admission, and 10 to 20% become delirious during hospitalization [53]. The incidence of postoperative delirium among patients ≥ 70y. is 15 to 25% after elective procedures and 35 to 65% after emergency and orthopedic procedures (eg, hip fracture repair).

Etiologically delirium in the elderly (especially in advanced age) develops as non-specific global brain reaction of transitory character to the numerous causal noxas. From the practical viewpoint the possible risk factors may be seen in three different causes: 1. factors on the patient's side (predisposing diseases); 2. acute disease; 3. iatrogenic and environmental reasons. Careful examination of the patient (including the case history) can possibly explain its cause. State of acute confusion may be induced usually both intracranially and extracranially (Figure n. 2)

Usual causes of delirium	
Intracranial	Extracranial
Infection (eg, meningitis, encephalitis) Seizure diseases, state after stroke Strokes Subdural hematoma Tumor Dementia, depresssion Psychiatric diseases	Anaesthesia State after neck hip fracture Hyperkapnia Hypotermia Hypoxia Infection (respiratory and urinary tract) Intoxication or abstinential syndrom (alcohol or addictive substances) Metabolic disturbances (eg, liver or renal failure, electrolyt disbalance, hyper- or hypoglycemia) Heart attack Psychologic and environmental changes
Any drugs generally	

Figure 2. Usual cause of delirium (intra- i extracranial).

Occurrence of delirium in ICU hospitalized patients vary from 20% [10], through 70% [72] to 80% [29] according to the type of patient set and used methodology of the assessment. In older people admitted at ICU it has close relation to the earlier present cognitive disorder or usage of artificial ventilation [82]. This can lead primarily in older persons with mental deterioration to complications as aspiration, nosocomial pneumonia, reintubation and selfextubation [90].

Peterson [80] describes in 613 patients treated at ICU in accordance with assessment of psychomotoric activity hyperactive delirium as rare (< 5%), whereas hypoactive type (often in older) and mixed delirium in majority of cases. Hypoactive kind [73] is dangerous at ICU and standard wards with risk to remain not be distinguished in more than 2/3 both doctors and nurses. In the elderly discovery of hypoactive delirium is often explained by dementia, depression or merely through hospitalization at ICU in elderly persons critically ill.

Delirium doubles the risk of mortality, institutionalization and decrease of functional activity during two years after discharge from hospital in patients, which were earlier fully self-sufficient [85].

SYMPTOMS AND SIGNS

A patient with delirium has acute fluctuations in mental status, with varying levels of inattention and altered levels of consciousness. Changes in orientation, memory, and abstract thinking may occur but are not diagnostic. Psychomotor activity (level of arousal) may be variably abnormal. Hallucinations, delusions, tremor, abnormalities in the sleep-wake cycle, and other symptoms may be present.

Dyspnoe, stenocardia, cyanosis or paresis at delirium may suggest real cause of the situation in cardiopulmonary or neurological region. In advanced age very essential dehydration can participate on confusional state.

DIAGNOSIS

Failure to diagnose or misdiagnosis occurs in up to 80% of cases but is less likely with interdisciplinary input (eg, from physicians, nurses, and persons who know the patient well, such as family members). The Confusion Assessment Method (CAM) scale may be the most useful tool for diagnosing delirium (table no. 3).

Table 3. Confusion Assessment Method (CAM) – Inouye

Sudden onset and fluctuating course 1*	0-4 p. total score
Vigilance disturbances (fatigue, inability of concentration) 1*	* essential for dg. delirium
Thinking disorders (incoherent, paralogical, volatile) 1	≥3 p. probably delirium
Consciousness disorders (agitation, somnolence, stupor, coma) 1	

Thorough history, physical examination and laboratory evaluation are important for the diagnosis.

According to clinical vision and particularly to psychomotoric activity we can in principle distinguish three types of delirium [73]:

- Hyperactive – about 15% connected with increased psychomotoric unrest which is relatively easily distinguishable. This accompany usually hallucinations, delusions.
- Hypoactive – about 20% in elderly more frequent and often could be overlooked. Patients are confused, letargic and have distinct defect of the attention.
- Mixed type – about 50% has fluctuating course between hyper- and hypoactive epizods

DIFFERENTIAL DIAGNOSIS

The primary differential diagnoses are depression and dementia, both of which may co-exist with delirium. Differentiation between delirium and dementia is not always clear, and the features of the two syndromes sometimes overlap. Onset of delirium is rapid; dementia usually develops slowly, although that one caused by a stroke or anoxia may occur acutely.

Complications

Patients with delirium are particularly vulnerable to iatrogenic problems, especially those due to physical or chemical (ie, drug) restraints. Bladder and bowel incontinence or retention is common and can directly contribute to delirium. Bedridden patients with delirium are prone to atelectasis, deconditioning, and pressure sores.

Prognosis and Treatment

Hospitalized patients with delirium [29,69,72] have up to a 10-fold higher risk of medical complications (including death), longer hospitalization, higher hospital costs, and increased need for postacute placement at discharge.

Behavioral control may be necessary to ensure patient´s comfort and to promote safety. Usually, social restraint is preferred to physical or chemical restraints.

A. Non-Specific Proceedings

- diagnosis and therapy possible *somatic disease* provoking delirium
- attention given to *hydration and realimentation*
- *stop taking psychoactive or other risky drugs*
- *environmental arrangement:* with eliminating possible stressors, patient's reassurance better in presence of known person (pertinently placement some things from home in patient's room) and permanent well-balanced quiet psychic stimulation.
- universally it is necessary to *emphasize installation of regular everyday regimen and professional monitoring, including patients´ reassurance.*
- *physical restraints* will be single possible solution of situation by agitated unrested patients who endanger themselves and environment. They will be used only temporarily before or after application of calming psychopharmac. Delirious seniors will need *permanent supervision.*

B. Specific Treatment

If non-pharmacologic management shown above at acute confusional state is not sufficiently effective and the reason of its development is not an organic cause, which would be treatable by drugs, thereafter specific therapy of the delirium is fully indicated [11,26,86]. Unrest and confusional state can provoke for example also inadequately inhibited pain mainly in patients with malignancies.

If the above mentioned symptoms (consciousness disturbance, unrest, confusion, hallucinations, aggressivity towards environment and her/himself too) are spreaded, if the patient disrupts coexistence in collective (nursing home etc.), ward's operation, and own safety and environment, it is the doctor's decision on usage of psychoactive drugs, physical restraints (including transfer to a closed psychiatric ward).

In simple cases it is possible to use sedatives from the group of benzodiazepins with strong anxiolytic and less calming effect, as oxazepam; chlordiazepoxid, alprazolam, klonazepam. As injection are for disposal im. or iv. in cases of enormous aggitation diazepam a clonazepam. From neuroleptics 1st generation is for usage melperon, which is on the market in both injection form and tablets. From the group of sedative neuroleptics haloperidol. deserves our attention, which is usable as injection also reapeatedly iv. or im. (for example every 6 hours, maximum day doses is 20 mg). Long-term peroral dosis of haloperidol is 0,5- 1 mg 3-times a day. Another very effective neuroleptic drug is risperidon, usually 0,25- 1 mg/day. Tiapridum from the group of atypical neuroreptics with high activity to dopamin D2 – receptors. It does not affect the formation extrapyramidal syndrome and also further subsidiary effect are in tiapridum less often expressed. All drugs used to treat agitation can produce oversedation (54,68), and their use sometimes prolongs delirium and increases the risk of complications.

Chapter 14

THERMOREGULATORY DISORDERS

Homeothermy is achieved in humans by the coordinated response of autonomic, metabolic, and behavioral activities integrated within CNS. Autonomic disorders in human thermoregulation, particularly in the more vulnerable elderly persons, can lead to the development of abnormal thermal conditions such as hypothermia and hyperthermia [21,53,79]. Moreover thermal perception deficit plays an important role in the elderly.

Diagnosis is usually clear from the history and physical examination. Core body temperature is measured rectally or esophageally using an electronic thermometer or a mercury thermometer with an extended lower and upper range.

EFFECTOR MECHANISMS OF THERMOREGULATION

In cold conditions, shivering and non-shivering thermogenesis operate to maintain deep body temperature in addition to vasoconstriction. Non-shivering thermogenesis in the adult human can be produced by the calorigenic action of catecholamines and other hormones such as thyreoid hormone. The facultative component of the thermogenic reaction depends on sympathetic nervous control and it has been shown to be significantly lower in elderly people. Noradrenergic vasoconstrictor neurons probably represent the largest group of sympathetic nerves supplying the skin and their dysfunction plays an important role in thermoregulatory lability of the elderly in cold conditions.

Vasodilatation in hot weather activates vasodilatator system in skin. The degree of thermally induced vasodilatation attained by the elderly is usually less than in younger people and corresponds to a reduced cardiac output. Marked regression of secretory cutaneous glands with age, together with a significant decrease in the number of immunoreactive sympathetic nerves.

HYPOTHERMIA

This is defined as the condition in which deep body temperature falls below 35^0 C, commonly arises as the result of accidental and excessive exposure to cold. Most of the latter cases appear to defend a lowered temperature set point by active body heat dissipation through vasodilatation and sweating and by decreasing heat generation by behavioral mechanisms.

Low deep body temperature is then associated with existing pathological conditions such as diabetes mellitus, Alzheimer disease, or the effect of medications (phenothiazines, hypnotics, anxiolytics, antidepressants, and alkohol abuse). Elderly people are susceptible to cold because of lower thermogenesis, reduced sympathetic vasoconstrictor activity, and blunted temperature perception and behavioral response to temperature change [60]. Though once considered to be a significant cause of winter mortality in advanced age in developed countries situated in the north. Hypothermia is known to cause about 600 deaths every year in the USA [22]. For elderly patients with diagnosed hypothermia, the mortality rate is 50%. Mortality rate increases with ageing, particularly after age 75.

Risk Factors for Hypothermia in the Elderly

- Reduced physical activity, immobility, dementia, undernutrition, many other common disorders, and many commonly used drugs.
- May not recognize that they are cold and may not shiver.
- Require more extensive routine laboratory testing than younger patients.
- Since hypothyroidism is common among the elderly, it should always be excluded as a cause or contributor.

Etiology

Most episodes of hypothermia are initiated outdoors by ambient temperatures < 15.5° C, but frail elderly people may become hypothermic while indoors at temperatures as warm as 22° to 24° C. Iatrogenic hypothermia can occur when unclothed elderly patients undergo surgery in a cool operating room.

Many age-related physiologic changes, including a diminished perception of cold, predispose elderly people to hypothermia [100]. Decreased responsiveness to endogenous catecholamines reduces the vasoconstrictor and shivering responses to cold. A decrease in lean body mass reduces the efficiency of shivering for producing heat. Reduced physical activity and caloric intake lower the metabolic rate, decreasing endogenous heat production.

Symptoms and Signs

Symptoms and signs of hypothermia are insidious and may be transient. Elderly people with a body temperature between 35° and 36.1° C often report feeling cold, but patients with lower body temperature usually do not feel this. Their skin has a cadaveric pallor and chill, and pressure points have erythematous, bullous, or purpuric patches. Shivering may not occur. Instead, marked rigidity develops accompanied by a generalized increase in muscle tone; occasionally, a fine tremor is present.

Neurologic findings include thick, slow speech and ataxic gait; deep tendon reflexes are depressed. Sleepiness and confusion may progress to coma.

Cardiovascular findings are tachycardia and elevated BP initially. Later on, hypotension and progressive sinus bradycardia occur. Cardiac arrest due to ventricular fibrillation or asystole is increasingly likely as body temperature falls to < 30° C.

GI findings can include abdominal distention, diminished or absent bowel sounds, and, less often, vomiting.

Diagnosis

Hypothermia is often and easily missed. Clinical findings are usually nonspecific and can suggest other disorders (e.g. MI, infection, hypoglycemia).

Laboratory testing should include CBC; platelet count; PT and PTT/INR; measurement of urea, creatinine, electrolyte, CPK, plasma glucose, and serum lipase and amylase levels; thyroid and liver function tests; AB gases; ECG; and chest and abdominal x-rays. Laboratory findings are usually nonspecific. Hemoconcentration, leukocytosis, acidosis, thrombocytopenia, and hyperglycemia are common.

Treatment

Hypothermia, even if mild, should be treated in the hospital, usually in an ICU. Treatment includes body warming and supportive measures for the complications of hypothermia. Most drugs are avoided as long as hypothermia is present. They are ineffective and poorly metabolized; as a result, enhanced and undesirable rebound effects may occur as patients are warmed. Because most patients are hypovolemic, IV fluids are given, usually 1 L of 0.9% normal saline solution warmed from 37° to 45° C.

In elderly patients, rapid warming with an external heat source is avoided if possible because it can lead to a syndrome of severe hypotension, new cardiac arrhythmias, and worsening metabolic abnormalities, culminating in death. Therefore, stable elderly patients are warmed by conserving endogenous heat production and minimizing external heat loss (passive warming) - a slow method. For passive warming, body temperature increases about 0.6° C/h. Room temperature is kept > 21.1° C, and blankets or more effective insulating materials are used to retain body heat.

Active external warming is in the elderly relatively contarindicated. If a body temperature is ≤ 30° C; in such cases, active external and active core warming is necessary. Otherwise in advanced age passive warming is suitable. If a nonperfusing cardiac rhythm (e.g. ventricular fibrillation, asystole) occurs at a temperature < 30° C, warming must occur as quickly as possible because, at such a temperature, the heart is unresponsive to electrical defibrillation and because drug therapy for most arrhythmias is ineffective.

Defibrillation may be attempted starting at 2 joules/kg. If a single stacked sequence (200/300/360 joules) is ineffective, further attempts are deferred until temperature increases. Resuscitation should be continued, and patients are not pronounced dead until temperature reaches 35° C, unless obviously lethal injuries or disorders are present.

Although hyperglycemia is common among patients with hypothermia, insulin is rarely given unless plasma glucose levels are > 400 mg/dL (> 22.2 mmol/L); insulin is ineffective at low temperatures. Production of endogenous insulin during warming may lead to hypoglycemia. Plasma glucose should be monitored regularly.

Prevention

When outdoors in cold weather, elderly people should wear several layers of warm clothing and protect themselves against moisture and wind. Gloves and socks should be kept as dry as possible. A warm head covering is particularly important because 30% of body heat is lost from the head.

Indoors, elderly people with risk factors for hypothermia should keep room temperatures ≥ 18.3° C. Adequate caloric intake and, if possible, exercise help sustain endogenous heat production. Drugs that increase risk should be stopped whenever possible.

HYPERTHERMIA

Hyperthermia is defined as an abnormally high body temperature due to inadequate or inappropriate responses of heat-regulating mechanisms.

About 80% of people who die of heatstroke are > 50. Also, the number of deaths resulting from majority of other disorders increases during hot, humid weather, particularly among the elderly. For example, deaths attributed to diabetes, pulmonary disorders, and hypertension increase by > 50% during heat waves. Elevation of deep body temperature above 38.4 C is arbitrarily considered to be hyperthermic condition.

HEAT EXHAUSTION

Heat exhaustion is a syndrome of weakness, malaise, nausea, and other non-specific symptoms caused by heat exposure; it is not life threatening. Thermoregulation is not impaired. Body temperature may be normal or increased up to 40° C.

Heat exhaustion results from depletion of fluids and electrolytes which may occur during exertion. Symptoms are non-specific and may not be recognized at first; they may include anorexia, thirst, nausea, vomiting, light-headedness, weakness, and muscle cramping.

Diagnosis

Diagnosis is through history and physical examination. In the elderly clinical status sometimes require IV fluid replacement (e.g. cardiac).

Treatment

Because elderly patients tend to present late and with severe symptoms (e.g. severe muscle cramping, syncope), treatment is usually IV administration of 0.9% normal saline solution. Volume and rate should be adjusted based on the patient's clinical response, and presence of heart failure, renal insufficiency or metabolic disorders.

Heat Stroke

Heatstroke [13] usually develops over days, usually during heat waves, and most often affects elderly people who do not have air conditioning. That causes multiple organ dysfunction and often death in advanced age.

Thermoregulatory autonomic impairment resulting in diminished sweating and peripheral vasodilatation is likely to be one of the factors that may lead to heat stroke in older people. In addition, factors controlling fluid balance, vasopressin‘s secretion and its renal response, and control of sodium balance are adversely affected by age. Commonly prescribed medications, anticholinergics, diuretics, and psychotropics increase the risk of heat intolerance in the elderly. Heat stroke is characterised by a deep body temperature > 40 C or more accompanied by CNS disturbances leading to convulsions and coma and anhidrosis, which is often present but is not pathognomic of the conditions. Heat-related death during urban heat waves, especially in the elderly population, are generally not directly due to thermoregulatory failure but often rather due to existing cardiovascular disease worsened by heat waves.

Etiology

Classical heatstroke occurs after days of heat exposure, typically during heat waves, and tends to affect sedentary, elderly people who do not have air conditioning and who have limited access to fluids. Risk factors for classical heatstroke in the elderly include low socioeconomic status, impaired self-care ability, alcoholism, other comorbid mental or physical disorders (e.g. cardiovascular or cerebrovascular disease, diabetes, COPD), and use of certain drugs. Overall, heatstroke occurs much more often in people > 65 than in younger people.

Pathophysiology

Organ dysfunction may involve the CNS, kidneys, lungs (acute respiratory distress syndrome), heart, coagulation system, and occasionally liver. In the brain, edema, patchy congestion, and diffuse petechial hemorrhages are common. Rhabdomyolysis can occur, resulting in acute renal failure. Aldosterone secretion may be increased. Lactate levels increase, resulting in metabolic acidosis and compensatory respiratory alkalosis. The coagulation cascade may become activated; rarely, full-blown disseminated intravascular coagulation results.

Symptoms and Signs

Heatstroke is characterized by a body temperature usually > 40° C and global brain dysfunction - eg, delirium, seizures, lethargy, stupor, coma [92]. Light-headedness, dizziness, headache, weakness, dyspnea, nausea, or loss of consciousness may precede development of full-blown heatstroke. Up to 20% of survivors have permanent brain damage. Renal insufficiency may become permanent, and body temperature may be labile for weeks. In elderly people with heatstroke, heart rate may be inappropriately slow despite hypovolemia.

Diagnosis

Case history matters and careful somatic examination (body temperature) is important. ECG (usually) shows changes in ST segments and T waves, premature ventricular contractions, supraventricular tachycardias, and conduction abnormalities [2,95]. What is important in laboratory findings is as follows:

- PT and PTT/INR: Elevated, often with a decreased fibrinogen level
- Electrolytes: Hypokalemia and high anion gap metabolic acidosis
- Urea and creatinine: Elevated
- CPK: Elevated, possibly reflecting rhabdomyolysis or cardiac muscle necrosis
- Liver function tests: Elevated transaminases or bilirubin
- Urinalysis by urethral catheter: Proteinuria

Treatment

Heatstroke is a medical emergency requiring immediate cooling measures [38]. Fanning the patient continuously while applying ice to the neck, axillae, and groin or while spraying the skin with cool water is usually effective. Cooling should be stopped when body temperature reaches about 38.8° C to avoid overcooling and hypothermia. Since heart failure or dehydration may occur and may be clinically unapparent central venous pressure monitoring to guide fluid replacement is also very suitable.

Prevention

Caregivers should be alert to symptoms of heatstroke in elderly people in very hot weather. Elderly people should wear light, porous clothing and keep their windows open at night and shaded during the day; adequate fluid intake (even when they are not thirsty) and avoidance of exercise are inevitable.

Chapter 15

CONCLUSION

Our long-term experience with multi-morbid old patients leads us to a conclusion that once the senior has been detected as critically ill and the therapy in ICU was after admission introduced it is desirable to consider carefully all further comorbidities and any other additional treatment regarding the aspect of drug interactions and side effects. Unfortunately in multi-morbid seniors polypharmacy is mostly an inevitable part of therapeutic procedures.

The approach to older patients should be consistently individualised. New diagnostic methods and therapeutic algorithms used in ICU together enable us to treat successfully also elderly multi-morbid patients admitted by intensivists. These modern iatrotechniques make possible also the treatment (including recovery) and protect self-sufficiency and preserve quality of life in the elderly being critically ill.

REFERENCES

[1] Adler J, Bachur RG, Brenner B, Darling RG, Dronen SC, Dyne P (eds.):Emergency Medicine – Medical Reference, e Medicine, from WebMD, 2006.

[2] Akhtar MJ, Al-Nozha M, Al-Harthi S, Nouh MS: Electrocardiographic abnormalities in patients with heat stroke. *Chest* 1993; 104: 411-414.

[3] Aronow W.S. : Effects of aging on the heart. In: Tallis R, Fillit H (eds.): *Brocklehurst's Textbook of Geriatric Medicine and* Gerontology 6th ed. London, Churchill Livingstone, 2003, 1478p..

[4] Asplund K, Gustafson Y, Jacobsson C et al.: Geriatric- Based Versus General Wards for Older Acute Medical Patients: A Randomized Comparison of Outcomes and Use of Resources. *JAGS* 48; 2000: 1381-1388

[5] Barba R, Martinez-Espinosa S, Rodriguez-Garcia E, et al. Poststroke dementia: clinical features and risk factors. *Stroke* 2000; 31: 1494-501.

[6] Bartke A, Brown-Borg H, Matison R, Kinney R, Hauck S, Wright C: Prolonged longevity of hypopituitary dwarf mice, *Exp.Gerontol.* 2001; 36: 21-28

[7] Beck LH: The aging kidney. Defending a delicate balance of fluid and electrolytes. *Geriatrics* 2000; 55: 26-32

[8] Beckman JA, Creager MA, Libby P. Diabetes and Atherosclerosis. Epidemiology, Pathophysiology, and Management. *JAMA* 2002; 287: 2570-81.

[9] Beers MH, Thomas VJ, Jones TV (eds.) (2006) The Merck Manual of Geriatrics- 7th edition, Merck and Co, NY, 2006, electronic version.

[10] Bergeron N, Dubois MJ, Dumont M, et al: Intensive Care Delirium Screening Checklist: evaluation of a new screening tool. *Intensive Care Med.* 2001; 27: 859-864.

[11] Blackburn JA, Dulmus CN (editors): Handbook of gerontology : evidence-based approaches to theory, practice, and policy , *Hoboken,* N.J. Wiley, NY, 2007, 566p.

[12] Bombard FS, Sue DY (eds.): Current Critical Care Diagnosis and Treatment, Second Edition, Lange Medical Books/McGraw-Hill Medical Publishing Division, New York, 2003.

[13] Bouchama A, Knochel JP: Heat stroke. *N. Engl. J. Med.* 2002; 346: 1978-1988.

[14] Brandes RP, Fleming I, Busee R: Endothelial aging. *Cardiovasc.Res.* 2005;66: 286-294.

[15] Braunwald E, Zipes DP, Libby P (eds.): Heart Disease, 6th edition – a Textbook of Cardiovascular Medicine, Philadelphia, *W.B.Saunders Comp.*, 2001, 2297 pp.

[16] Brodde OE, Lineweber K: Autonomic receptor systems in the failing and aging heart: similarities and differences. *Eur. J. Pharmacol.* 2004; 500: 167-176.

[17] Brunner-Ziegler S, Heinze G, Ryffel M, Kompatscher M, Slany J, Valentin A: "Oldest old" patients in intensive care: prognosis and therapeutic activity. *Wien Klin Wochenschr.* 2007; 119: 14-19.

[18] Burns E, Goodwin JS: Immunology of Aging in Geriatric Medicíně. In: Cassel ChK, Cohen HJ Larson EB et al. (eds.): Geriatric Medicine/ thirtd ed. New York, *Springer*, 1997, 1200p.

[19] Buttler G: Increasing life expectancy - what are the promises of demography? *Z Gerontol Geriat*, 36; 2003: 90-94 (in German).

[20] Campbell AJ, Cook JA, Adey G, Cuthbertson BH: Predicting death and readmission after intensive care discharge. *Br. J. Anaesth.* 2008;100: 656-562.

[21] Cassel ChK, Cohen HJ Larson EB et al. (eds.): Geriatric Medicine/ thirtd ed. New York, *Springer*, 1997, 1200p.

[22] Center for Disease Control: Hypothermia-related deaths-January 1996-December 1997, and United States, 1979-1995. *MMWR Morb. Mortal Wkly. Rep.* 1998; 47: 1037-1040.

[23] Connolly M: Age-related changes in the respiratory system. In: Tallis R, Fillit H (eds.): Brocklehurst's Textbook of Geriatric Medicine and Gerontology 6th ed. London, *Churchill Livingstone*, 2003, 1478p.

[24] Cook D J, Rook GA: Priorities in perioperative geriatrics. *Anesth. Anlg.* 2003; 96: 1823-1836.

[25] Coschigano KT, Clemmons D, Blush LL, Kopchick JJ: Assessment of growth parameters and life span of GHR/BP gene disrupted mice. *Endokrinology* 2000; 141: 2608-2613

[26] Devlin JW, Holbrook AM, Fuller HD: The effect of ICU sedation guidelines and pharmacist interventions on clinical outcomes and drug cost. *Ann. Pharmacother.* 1997; 31: 689-695.

[27] Dowdy DW, Eid MP, Sedrakyan A, Mendez-Tellez PA, Pronovost PJ, Herridge MS, Needham DM: Quality of life in adult survivors of critical illness: a systematic review of the literature. *Intensive Care Med.* 2005; 31: 611-620.

[28] Duthie EH, Katz PR and Malone ML (eds.): The practice of geriatrics 4th ed., Philadelphia: *Saunders Elsevier,* 2007, 681p.

[29] Ely EW, Inouye SK, Bernard GR, et al: Delirium in mechanically ventilated patients: Validity and reliability of the confusion assessment method for the intensive care unit (CAM-ICU). *JAMA* 2001; 286: 2703-2710.

[30] Feldman M, Friedman LS, Sleisenger MH (eds).Sleisenger and Fordtran's g astrointestinal and Liver Disease, 7. ed. Philadelphia, *Saunders,* 2002.

[31] Ferrari AU, Radaelli A, Centolla M: Aging and the cardiovascular system. *J. Appl. Physiol.* 2003; 95: 2591-2597.

[32] Fortin M, Bravo G, Hudon G, Vanasse A, Lapointe L: Prevalence of Multi-morbidity Among Adults Seen in Family Praktice. *Annals of Family Medicine* 2005; 3: 223-228.

[33] Fried LP, Borhani NO, Enright P, Furberg CD, Gardin JM, Kronmal RA, Kuller LH, Manolio TA, Mittelmark MB, Newman A, et al.: The Cardiovascular Health Study: design and rationale. *Ann. Epidemiol.* 1991;1: 263-276.

[34] Fried LP, Hadley EC, Walston JD, Newman AB, Guralnik JM, Studenski S, Harris TB, Ershler WB, Ferrucci L: From bedside to bench: research agenda for frailty. *Sci. Aging Knowledge Environ.* 2005; 31: pe24.

[35] Friedman SM, Steinwachs DM, Temkin-Greener H, Mukamel DB: Informal caregivers and the risk of nursing home admission among individuals enrolled in the program of all-inclusive care for the elderly. *Gerontologist.* 2006; 46: 456-463.

[36] Friedman SM, Mendelson DA, Kates SL, McCann RM: Geriatric co-management of proximal femur fractures: total quality management and protocol-driven care result in better outcomes for a frail patient population. *J. Am. Geriatr. Soc.* 2008; 56: 1349-1356.

[37] Frost SA, Alexandrou E, Bogdanovski T, Salamonson Y, Davidson PM, Parr MJ, Hillman KM: Severity of illness and risk of readmission to intensive care: a meta-analysis. *Resuscitation.* 2009; 80:505-510.

[38] Gaffin SL, Gardner JW, Flinn SD: Cooling methods for heatstroke victims. *Ann. Intern. Med.* 2000; 132: 678.

[39] Gammack JK and Morley JE (eds.): Geriatric medicine, Philadelphia : *Saunders*, 2006

[40] Gerbes AL, Gülberg V, Bilzer M et al. Evaluation of serum cystatin C concentration as a marker of renal function in patients with cirrhosis of the liver. *Gut.* 2002; 50: 106–110.

[41] Goldmann L, Bennett JC (eds.): Cecil Textbook of Medicine. 21st Edition. Philadelphia, *W. B. Saunders Comp.*, 2000, 2308p.

[42] Gupta Abhaya: Measurement scales used in elderly care / Abhaya Gupta ; forewords by Jeremy Playfer and Bim Bhowmick OBE, Oxford : Radcliffe Publishing, 2008

[43] Hall JB, Schmidt GA, Wood LDH et al.(eds). Principles of Critical Care. care.3. ed., McGraw-Hill, Medical Publishing Division , New York 2005.

[44] Hazzard WR: Scientific progress in geriatric syndromes: earning an "A" on the 2007 report card on academic geriatrics. *J. Am. Geriatr. Soc.* 2007; 55: 794-796.

[45] Heltweg B: Antitumor Activity of a Small-Molecule Inhibitor of Human Silent Information Regulator 2 Enzymes. *Cancer Research* 2006; 66: 4368-4377

[46] Hirokawa K: Immunity and Ageing. In: Pathy M.S. John, Sinclair Alan J., Morley John E. (eds.): Principles and practice of geriatric medicine, 4th ed., Chichester : *Wiley*, 2006.

[47] Humes D (ed. in chief): Kelley's Textbook of Internal Medicine. Philadelphia, Lippincott Williams and Wilkins, 2000, 3254s.

[48] Hunter JA, Haslett C, Chilver AR, Boon NA, Colledge A (eds.): Davidson's Principle and Practice of Medicine. 19th Edition. Edinburgh, *Churchill Livingstone*, 2002, 1296p.

[49] Inouye SK, Studenski S, Tinetti ME, Kuchel GA: Geriatric syndromes: clinical, research, and policy implications of a core geriatric concept. *J. Am. Geriatr. Soc.* 2007; 55: 780-791.

[50] Inzerillo A, Iqbal J, Troen B, Meier DE: Skeletal fragility. In: Cassel ChK, Cohen HJ Larson EB et al. (eds.): Geriatric Medicine/ thirtd ed. New York, *Springer,* 1997, 1200p.

[51] Jassal SV, Oreoupoulos DG: Aging and the urinary tract. In Tallis R, Fillit H (eds.): Brocklehurst's Textbook of Geriatric Medicine and Gerontology 6th ed. London, *Churchill Livingstone*, 2003, 1478p.

[52] Kalvach Z., Zadák Z, Jirák R, Zavázalová H.,Sucharda P. a kol Geriatrie a gerontologie, Grada Publishing a.s., Praha, 2004, 961s.

[53] Kasper DL, Fauci AS, Longo DL, Braunwald E, Hauser SL, Jameson JL (eds.): Harrison's Principles of Internal Medicine 16th Edition, McGraw-Hill Medical Publishing Division, New York, 2005.

[54] Katzung Bertram, G. (ed.): Basic and Clinical Pharmacology. San Francisco, McGraw- Hill Professional Publishing, 2003, 1088 p.

[55] Kaufman, H.., Biaggioni, I.: Disorders of the autonomic nervous system. Tallis R, Fillit H (eds.): Brocklehurst's Textbook of Geriatric Medicine and Gerontology 6th ed. London, *Churchill Livingstone*, 2003, 1478p.

[56] Kelleher, C.L.: Disorders of water and electrolyte metabolism. In: Tallis R, Fillit H (eds.): Brocklehurst's Textbook of Geriatric Medicine and Gerontology 6th ed. London, *Churchill Livingstone*, 2003, 1478p.

[57] Kellum JA, Song M, Venkataraman R: Effects of hyperchloremic acidosis on arterial pressure and circulating inflammatory molecules in experimental sepsis. *Chest* 2004; 125: 243-248.

[58] Khaw KT: How many, how old, how soon *BMJ* 1997; 319: 1350-1352.

[59] Kimball's biology page www.users.rcn.com/jkimball.ma.ultranet/ biologypages/W/welcome/hml, 2008.

[60] Koutsavlis AT, Kosatsky T: Environmental-temperature injury in a Canadian metropolis. *J. Environ. Health.* 2003; 66: 40-45.

[61] Kriška M (ed.): Memorix klinickej farmakológie. Kriška M (ed.): Memorix of clinical pharmacology. Bratislava, Slovak Academic Press, 2002, 879s.

[62] Kuntz E, Kuntz HD. Hepatology : Principles and practice,, history, morphology, biochemistry, diagnostics, clinic, therapy. Heidelberg, *Springer*, 2006.

[63] Lakatta E: Aging and Cardiovascular System. In: Beers MH, Thomas VJ, Jones TV (eds.): The Merck Manual of Geriatrics- 7th edition, Merck and Co, NY, 2006, electronic version.

[64] Lamb JF, Morley JE: The pituitary gland. In: Pathy M.S. John, Sinclair Alan J., Morley John E. (eds.): Principles and practice of geriatric medicine, 4th ed., Chichester : *Wiley*, 2006.

[65] Leng SX, Xue QL, Tian J, Walston JD, Fried LP: Inflammation and frailty in older women. *J. Am. Geriatr. Soc.* 2007; 55: 864-871.

[66] Lincová D, Farghali H (eds.): Základní a aplikovaná farmakologie. Praha, *Galén- Karolinum*, 2002, 601s.

[67] Lipsitz, L.A.: Orthostatic Hypotension. In: Beers MH, Thomas VJ, Jones TV (eds.): The Merck Manual of Geriatrics- 7th edition, Merck and Co, NY, 2006, electronic version.

[68] Lüllmann H, Mohr K, Wehling M (Ed.): Farmakologie a toxikologie. Praha, Grada Publishing, 2002, 694s.

[69] Marcantonio ER, Flacker JM, Wright RJ, Resnick NM: Reducing delirium after hip fracture: a randomized trial. *J. Am. Geriatr. Soc.* 2001; 49: 516-522.

[70] Masoro EJ and Austad SN (editors): Handbook of the biology of aging, 6th ed., Burlington, MA; London: Elsevier Academic Press, 2006, 660p.

[71] McDowell Anderson, W., Tockman, M.S.: Aging and the lungs In: Beers MH, Thomas VJ, Jones TV (eds.): The Merck Manual of Geriatrics- 7th edition, Merck and Co, NY, 2006, electronic version.

[72] McNicoll L, Pisani MA, Zhang Y, et al: Delirium in the intensive care unit: occurrence and clinical course in older patients. *J. Am. Geriatr. Soc.* 51:591, 2003.

[73] Meagher DJ, Trzepacz PT: Motoric subtypes of delirium. *Semin. Clin. Neuropsychiatry* 5:75, 2000.

[74] Moody HR: Aging : concepts and controversies, 5th ed., Thousand Oaks, Calif. ; London : *Pine Forge*, c2006

[75] Morley JE, Kim MJ: Endocrinology of Aging. In: Pathy M.S. John, Sinclair Alan J., Morley John E. (eds.): Principles and practice of geriatric medicine, 4th ed., Chichester : *Wiley*, 2006.

[76] Muller M, van den Beld AW, van der Schouw YT, Grobbee DE and Lamberts SWJ: Effects of Dehydroepiandrosterone and Atamestane Supplementation on Frailty in Elderly Men. *J. Clin. Endocrinol. Metab.* 2006; 91: 3988-3991.

[77] Nikolaus T (Hrsg.): Klinische Geriatrie, Berlin, *Springer* 2000, 1105p.

[78] Oskvig RM: Special problems in the elderly. *Chest* 1999; 115: 158-164.

[79] Pathy M.S. John, Sinclair Alan J., Morley John E. (eds.): Principles and practice of geriatric medicine, 4th ed., Chichester : *Wiley*, 2006.

[80] Peterson JF, Truman BL, Shintani A, et al: The prevalence of hypoactive, hyperactive, and mixed type delirium in medical ICU patients. *J. Am. Geriatr. Soc.* 2003; 51: S174.

[81] Pirlich M, Schütz T, Norman K, Gastell S, Lübke HJ, Bischoff SC, Bolder U, Frieling T, Güldenzoph TH, Hahn K, Jauch KW, Schindler K, Stein J, Volkert D, Weimann A, Werner JJ, Wolf C, Zürcher G, Bauer P, Lochs H: German hospital malnutrition study. *Clinical Nutrition* 2006; 5: 563-572.

[82] Pisani MA, McNicoll L, Inouye SK: Cognitive impairment in the intensive care unit. *Clin. Chest Med.* 2003; 24: 727-737.

[83] Rai Gurcharan S and Mulley GP (eds.): Elderly medicine : a training guide, 2nd ed., Edinburgh, *Churchill Livingstone Elsevier*: 2007.

[84] Randers E, Ivarsen P, Erlandsen EJ et al. Plasma cystatin C as a marker of renal function in patients with liver cirrhosis. *Scand. J. Clin. Lab. Invest.* 2002; 62: 129–134.

[85] Ranhoff AH, Rozzini R, Sabatini T, Cassinadri A, Boffelli S, Trabucchi M: Delirium in a subintensive care unit for the elderly: occurrence and risk factors. *Aging Clin. Exp. Res.* 2006; 18: 440-445.

[86] Ratnaike RN (ed.). Practical Guide to Geriatric Medicine. New York: *Mc Graw Hill Comp., Inc.*, 2002, 958p.

[87] Rhee MK, Ziemer DC, Kolm P, Philips LS: Postchallenge glucose rises with increasing age even when glucose tolerance is normal. *Diabetic Medicine* 2006; 23: 1174-1179.

[88] Rivera-Fernandez R, Navarrete-Navarro P, Fernandez-Mondejar E, Rodriguez-Elvira M, Guerrero-Lałpez F, Vazquez-Mata G; Project for the Epidemiological Analysis of Critical Care Patients (PAEEC) Group: Six-year mortality and quality of life in critically ill patients with chronic obstructive pulmonary disease. *Crit. Care. Med.* 2006; 34: 2317-2324.

[89] Rivera-Fernandez R, Sanchez-Cruz JJ, Abizanda-Campos R, Vazquez-Mata G: Quality of life before intensive care unit admission and its influence on resource utilization and mortality rate. *Crit. Care Med.* 2001; 29: 1701-1709.

[90] Roberts JR, Hedges JR: Clinical Procedures in Emergency Medicine, 4th ed., *Saunders, An Imprint of Elsevier*, NY, 2004.

[91] Rockwood K, Hubbard R: Frailty and the geriatrician. *Age Ageing*. 2004 Sep;33(5):429-430.

[92] Rosenberg H: Malignant hyperthermia. Available at: www.mhaus.org. Accessed June 3, 2004.

[93] Roubenoff R, Hughes VA: Sarcopenia: Current Concepts. *J. Gerontology*. 2000; 55: 716-724.

[94] Roubenoff R: Sarcopenia and its implications for the elderly. *European J. of Clinical Nutrition* 2000; 54: 40-47.

[95] Rousseau J-M, Villevieille T, Schiano P, et al: Reversible myocardial dysfunction after exertional heatstroke. *Intensive Care Med.* 2001; 27: 328-329.

[96] Salvedt I, Ophdal Mo E-S, Fayers P et al.: Reduced Mortality in Treating Acutely Sick, Frail Older Patients in a Geriatric Evaluation and Management Unit, A Prospective Randomized Trial. *JAGS*, 50, 2002; 5: 792-798.

[97] Sasajima Y, Sasajima T, Uchida H et al. Postoperative delirium in patients with chronic lower limb ischemia: what are the specific markers? *Eur. J. Vasc. Endovasc. Surg.* 2000; 20: 132-7.

[98] Scherl H: Increasing life expectancy – the big social issue of the 21st century? *Z Gerontol Geriat*, 36; 2003: 95-103 (in german).

[99] Seitz M: A long life – a wish and its limits. Aging with dignity and meaning. *Z Gerontol Geriat*, 36; 2003: 104- 109 (in german).

[100] Silfvast T, Pettila V: Outcome from severe accidental hypothermia in Southern Finland-A 10-year review. *Resuscitation* 2003; 59: 285-290.

[101] Sinclair AJ, Croxon SCM: Diabetes mellitus. In: Tallis R, Fillit H (eds.): Brocklehurst's Textbook of Geriatric Medicine and Gerontology 6th ed. London, Churchill Livingstone, 2003, 1478p.

[102] Sinclair AJ, Finucane P (eds.): Diabetes in Old Age. second edition. New York, *John Wiley and Sons*, 2001, 274 p.

[103] Solomon DH: Thyroid Disorders. In: In: Beers MH, Thomas VJ, Jones TV (eds.): The Merck Manual of Geriatrics- 7th edition, Merck and Co, NY, 2006, electronic version.

[104] Soriano RP, Fernandez HM, Cassel ChK, Leipzig R (eds.): Fundamentals of geriatric medicine : a case-based approach, New York : *Springer*, 2007.

[105] Stone CK, Humphries R (eds.): Current Emergency Diagnosis and Treatment 5th Edition, McGraw-Hill Companies, Inc., NY, 2004.

[106] Szanton SL, Seplaki CL, Thorpe RJ Jr, Allen JK, Fried LP: Socioeconomic status is associated with frailty: the Women's Health and Aging Studies. *J. Epidemiol. Community Health.* 2010; 64: 63-67.

[107] Tallis R, Fillit H (eds.): Brocklehurst's Textbook of Geriatric Medicine and Gerontology 6th ed. London, Churchill Livingstone, 2003, 1478s.

[108] Tariq SH: Gastrointestinal bleeding. In: Pathy M.S. John, Sinclair Alan J., Morley John E. (eds.): Principles and practice of geriatric medicine, 4th ed., Chichester : *Wiley*, 2006.

[109] Terry, B.P.: Aging and the lunte. In: Beers MH, Thomas VJ, Jones TV (eds.): The Merck Manual of Geriatrics- 7th edition, Merck and Co, NY, 2006, electronic version.

[110] Tintinalli JE, Kelen GD, Stapczynski JS (eds.). Emergency Medicine: A Comprehensive Study Guide 6th ed. , McGraw-Hill Medical Publishing Division, New York, 2004.

[111] Tintinalli JE, Kelen GD, Stapczynski JS (eds.): Emergency Medicine: A Comprehensive Study Guide - sixth edition , McGraw-Hill Medical Publishing Division , New York , 2004.

[112] Topinková E. Geriatrie pro praxi. Praha: *Galén*, 2005.

[113] Veldhuis JD, Bowers CY: Human GH pulsatility, an ensemble property regulated by age and gender. *J. of Endocrinological Investigation* 2003; 26: 799-813

[114] Walston J, Hadley EC, Ferrucci L, Guralnik JM, Newman AB, Studenski SA, Ershler WB, Harris T, Fried LP: Research agenda for frailty in older adults: toward a better understanding of physiology and etiology: summary from the American Geriatrics Society/National Institute on Aging Research Conference on Frailty in Older Adults. *J. Am. Geriatr. Soc.* 2006; 54: 991-1001.

[115] Wawruch M, Zikavska M, Wsolova L, Jezova D, Fialova D, Kunzo M, Kuzelova M, Lassanova M, Kruty P, Kriska M: Perception of potentially inappropriate medication in elderly patients by Slovak physicians. *Pharmacoepidemiol Drug Saf.* 2006; 15: 829-834

[116] Webster JR: Pulmonary Disease in Geriatric Medicine. Cassel ChK, Cohen HJ Larson EB et al. (eds.): Geriatric Medicine/ thirtd ed. New York, *Springer*, 1997, 1200p

[117] Williams ME: Geriatric physical diagnosis : a guide to observation and assessment, Jefferson, N.C. : McFarland and Co., c2008.

[118] Wilson MMG: Liver and gall bladder. In: Pathy M.S. John, Sinclair Alan J., Morley John E. (eds.): Principles and practice of geriatric medicine, 4th ed., Chichester : *Wiley*, 2006.

[119] Woodford,H: Essential geriatrics, Abingdon: *Radcliffe*, 2007.

[120] Woodhouse KW, O'Mahony MS: Frailty and ageing. *Age Ageing*. 1997; 26: 245-246.

[121] Yaffe K, Haan M, Blackwell T, Cherkasova E, Whitmer RA, West N: Metabolic syndrome and cognitive decline in elderly Latinos: findings from the Sacramento Area Latino Study of Aging study. *J. Am. Geriatr. Soc.* 2007; 55: 758-762.

INDEX

A

B

C

D

E

F

G

L

M

N

O

V

W

X

Y